Young People

and Substance Misuse

Young People and Substance Misuse

Edited by Ilana B. Crome, Hamid Ghodse,
Eilish Gilvarry and Paul McArdle

Gaskell

British Library Cataloguing-in-Publication Data
A catalogue record for this book is available from the British Library.
ISBN 1-904671-01-2

Distributed in North America
by Balogh International Inc.

The views presented in this book do not necessarily reflect
those of the Royal College of Psychiatrists, and the publishers
are not responsible for any error of omission or fact.

The Royal College of Psychiatrists is a registered charity (no. 228636).

The publishers have been unable to locate the copyright holder for table 12.1 (p. 164);
any reader with information on this matter should contact the Head of Publications at
the Royal College of Psychiatrists.

Printed in Great Britain by Bell & Bain Limited, Thornliebank, Glasgow

For our children –
Benjamin, Amir-Hossein, Nasreen, Ali-Reza, Áine and Tom

Contents

Contributors

Sue Bailey, Honorary Professor, Faculty of Postgraduate Health, University of Central Lancashire

Jane Christian, Service Manager, Turning Point, Druglink, Stoke-on-Trent, Staffordshire

Ilana B. Crome, Academic Director of Psychiatry and Professor of Addiction Psychiatry, University of Keele

Martin Frischer, Department of Medicines Management, University of Keele

Hamid Ghodse, Professor of Psychiatry and Addictive Behaviour, International Centre for Addiction Studies, St George's Hospital Medical School, London

Eilish Gilvarry, Centre for Alcohol and Drug Studies, Newcastle upon Tyne

Carole A. Kaplan, Senior Lecturer and Consultant in Child and Adolescent Psychiatry, St George's Hospital, Morpeth, Northumberland

Mervyn London, Brookfields Hospital, Cambridge

John Macleod, Department of Primary Care and General Practice, University of Birmingham

Ruth Marshall, Consultant Child and Adolescent Psychiatrist, Winnicott Centre, Manchester

Paul McArdle, Fleming Nuffield Unit, Department of Child Health, University of Newcastle upon Tyne

Daphne Rumball, Consultant in Addictions Psychiatry, The Bure Centre, Norfolk Mental Health Care Trust, Norwich

Richard Williams, Professor of Mental Health Strategy, University of Glamorgan and Consultant Child and Adolescent Psychiatrist, Gwent Health Care NHS Trust

Kate Woodhouse, Bristol

Acknowledgements

We would like to thank Dave Jago and the staff at Gaskell for their wise guidance at all stages from the initial proposal to completion.

The meticulous secretarial and administrative assistance in the collation of material by Marion Riley and Corrina Knight is greatly appreciated.

Preface

The foundations of adult health are laid during childhood and adolescence. As a child grows and matures there are ongoing transitions, during which major health and development needs evolve. Concurrently there are the challenges relating to these changes. The child and later the young person needs to learn how to handle and cope with these developments. The individual faces biological and psychological change. Social influences encompass role changes and extended expectations engendered by the transition into adulthood. There is then a more complex world, and one that is generally less stable and more volatile than that of the earlier phases of growth.

During all the stages from neonate to child and to adolescent, there is the need for a supportive, healthy and secure environment in which to grow and develop to the individual's full potential. One of the major threats during the latter stages is substance misuse. This may be precipitated by familial conflict and disruption, by unavoidable loss or by an undermining of the young person's sense of self – of a defined and understood identity. In some communities structures exist that are able to support vulnerable young people, but in modern industrial societies these structures have largely been eroded and the threats to stability are, therefore, heightened.

The relationship between dysfunction and substance misuse among young people has not received adequate attention. This state of affairs becomes even more disconcerting when we realise that these children and young people constitute nearly 40% of the world population. However, there is a vast reservoir of knowledge about the developmental process in all spheres of health in this age group. The vulnerability of children and adolescents to a catalogue of diseases and health problems, such as infectious disease and malnutrition, is well documented. Indeed, the level of childhood mortality, as an indicator of development and progress, illustrates the lack of health equity between various communities. The control of traditional 'disease' appears to be more attainable than the control of behavioural problems. In fact, there is now a belated but growing recognition that the proportion of children and adolescents with mental and behavioural problems has increased and that this group is likely to be particularly vulnerable. One example is the misuse of various psychoactive substances – both illicit drugs and alcohol and tobacco – which challenges the health and development of teenagers.

Information on and insight into the multiple effects of substances on mental state and physical well-being are steadily accumulating. Intoxication, for example, will increase the risk of accidental injury and engagement in unsafe sexual practices, which may lead to infection with HIV or hepatitis, or unintended pregnancy. Despite this 'new' knowledge and awareness, the interrelationship between the two has not been adequately studied. This is partly because substance misuse in adolescents is often considered a passing phase, when the misuse is 'recreational' or 'experimental' rather than 'problematic'. However, since substance misuse may delay growth and maturity, it is important to recognise the cumulative impact of interference with the developmental process. Gains or losses at any stage during this period may affect a young individual's health at a later stage, and may even affect the well-being of the next generation.

Although it is recognised that the provision of a healthier environment is bedevilled with more difficulties than was previously realised, and that the sociocultural control of behaviour is less predictable, it is important to realise that substance misuse is one of the most readily preventable conditions, especially among people in their teens and early adulthood. However, concurrent with the considerable consensus of disquiet about the increased misuse of substances by young people is the acceptance that there is a substantial gap in the implementation of available expertise to curtail such behaviour.

With this in mind, colleagues in various health and behavioural science disciplines have collated and integrated up-to-date information from research and clinical observations. It is hoped that all health care professionals as well as educationalists involved in the prevention of health problems and other consequences of substance misuse at this age will find it useful. The aim has been to make the book accessible not only to health professionals, but also to youth leaders, teachers, and social and other care workers. Further, it is addressed to a concerned and interested public, and not least to teenagers themselves. The authors and editors, led by Ilana Crome, have made every attempt to avoid the use of technical terms without losing the scientific basis and meaning of the issues under consideration. It is hoped that the text will contribute to the development of and practices and delivery of health care services in general and in particular to the prevention (or at least reduction) of psychoactive substance use among young people.

Hamid Ghodse

CHAPTER 1

Introduction

Hamid Ghodse

Key points

- The United Nations Convention on the Rights of the Child emphasises the need to protect children from illicit drug use and to prevent the use of children in illicit drug production and trafficking.
- There are many different definitions of the term 'young people', most of them related to the minimum age for particular activities.
- The criteria for the diagnosis of substance misuse and harmful use are derived from ICD–10 and DSM–IV.
- The reasons for drug use by young people include curiosity, rebellion, self-treatment of psychiatric symptoms, and peer pressure.
- The prevalence of drug taking among young people in the UK has increased over the past 20 years and the average age of first use is falling.
- Conduct and emotional disorders are risk factors for substance misuse in young people. Protective factors include a warm and happy family, high-achieving role models and an environment that encourages a healthy lifestyle.

Introduction

This chapter provides some background to the problem of substance misuse by young people, including aspects of epidemiology, the difficulties associated with defining what is meant by 'young people' and the principal contributory factors. In large part it cuts across the specific themes in other chapters, providing an introduction that it is hoped will facilitate a better understanding of the book as a whole.

The United Nations 1989 Convention on the Rights of the Child states that:

'Parties shall take all appropriate measures, including legislative, administrative, social and educational measures, to protect children from the illicit use of narcotic drugs and psychotropic substances as defined in the relevant international treaties, and to prevent the use of children in the illicit production and the trafficking of such substances.'

Many substances are controlled under international treaties. They can be broadly classified as follows:

- opium, morphine and other alkaloids, plus synthetic opioids;
- coca leaves and cocaine;
- cannabis products;
- other psychotropic substances that are misused or produce a state of dependence.

In addition, there are other drugs that are used by children that can affect their state of mind, damage their health or lead to dependence. These include substances such as alcohol, tobacco and solvents, the use of which by children is illegal in many countries by virtue of local legislation designed to protect them.

However, during the last decades of the twentieth century the use of and dependence on psychoactive drugs, including alcohol and nicotine, increased in many countries. The recreational use of drugs by young people, which contributed to the increase, was not a new phenomenon, but this experimental use of drugs for pleasure had never before involved so many young people and such a wide variety of drugs. Furthermore, the age at which drug users present for treatment has fallen (Sondhi *et al*, 1999). Illicit drug use and associated problems among young people, especially teenagers, received specific attention in the government strategy document *Tackling Drugs to Build a Better Britain* (Cabinet Office, 1998), which identified the prevention of illicit drug use among young people as a priority.

Definitions

In the UK, there is a confusing plethora of definitions of 'young people', according to the issue that is being discussed. For example, the age of criminal responsibility is 10 years; at 16 years of age, young people may purchase cigarettes (legally), have sex, get married and hold a driving licence for a motorcycle; at 17 years, they can have a driving licence for a car and join the armed forces; but they have to wait until they are 18 years before they can purchase alcohol (legally) and vote in elections. This book focuses on substance misuse by those under the age of 18 years, and all use of substances by people in this age group is considered misuse. The term 'drug misuse' is used interchangeably with 'substance misuse' and encompasses alcohol, tobacco and solvents as well as conventional pharmaceutical products and illicitly manu-factured substances.

Table 1.1 Criteria for substance abuse (DSM–IV) and harmful use (ICD–10)

DSM–IV	ICD–10
(A) A maladaptive pattern of substance use leading to clinically significant impairment or distress, as manifested by one (or more) of the following occurring within a 12-month period:	(A) A pattern of psycho-active substance use that is causing damage to health; the damage may be to physical or mental health
(1) Recurrent substance use resulting in a failure to fulfil major role obligations at work, school, or home (2) Recurrent substance abuse in situations that are physically hazardous (3) Recurrent substance-abuse-related legal problems (4) Continued substance abuse despite having persistent or recurrent social or interpersonal problems caused or exacerbated by the effects of the substance	
(B) Has never met the criteria for substance dependence for this class of substance	

Tables 1.1 and 1.2 outline the criteria in DSM–IV (*Diagnostic and Statistical Manual of Mental Disorders*) (American Psychiatric Association, 1994) and ICD–10 (*International Classification of Diseases*) (World Health Organization, 1992) that must be met before the diagnosis of a substance-related disorder (i.e. misuse, harmful use or dependence) can be made.

Reasons for drug use by young people

Adolescence is, of course, an age for curiosity and experimentation, and the inclusion of drug taking in this exploratory phase can be perceived as natural and normal. Risk taking, which can be thrilling, may provide further motivation. However, it is also a period of emotional upheaval and, for many, a period of intense emotional stress, as they progress from the safety and dependence of childhood to the independence of maturity. For example, early sexual activity is often perceived by adolescents as a source of pride and pleasure, but in practice is something many ill-prepared youngsters find unsatisfactory and which may further undermine their confidence. Because it is a time of such rapid change and stress, it is perhaps not surprising that adolescence is associated with psychological morbidity and that many adolescents seek to relieve their very real feelings of anxiety and depression by self-medication with widely available psychoactive drugs, just as many adults do. Smoking, drinking and taking drugs may also be perceived as 'adult' behaviours and therefore ones that an adolescent may feel under

Table 1.2 Criteria for dependence syndrome in DSM–IV and ICD–10

DSM–IV	ICD–10
(A) Diagnosis of dependence should be made if three (or more) of the following have been experienced or exhibited at any time in the same 12-month period:	(A) Diagnosis of dependence should be made if three or more of the following have been experienced or exhibited at some time during the past year:
(1) Tolerance defined by either need for a markedly increased amount of the substance to achieve intoxication or desired effect or a markedly diminished effect with continued use of the same amount of the substance	(1) A strong desire or sense of compulsion to take the substance
(2) Withdrawal as evidenced by either of the following: the characteristic withdrawal syndrome for the substance; or the same (or closely related) substance is taken to relieve or avoid withdrawal	(2) Difficulties in controlling substance-taking behaviour in terms of its onset, termination, or levels of use
(3) The substance is often taken in larger amounts over a longer period of time than was intended	(3) Physiological withdrawal state when substance use has ceased or been reduced, as evidenced by either of the following: the characteristic withdrawal syndrome for the substance; or use of the same (or closely related) substance with the intention of relieving or avoiding withdrawal symptoms
(4) Persistent desire or repeated unsuccessful efforts to cut down or control substance use	(4) Evidence of tolerance, such that increased doses of the psychoactive substance are required in order to achieve effects originally produced by lower doses
(5) A great deal of time is spent in activities necessary to obtain the substance, use the substance, or recover from its effects	(5) Progressive neglect of alternative pleasures or interests because of psychoactive substance use and increased amount of time necessary to obtain or take the substance or to recover from its effects
(6) Important social, occupational, or recreational activities given up or reduced because of substance use	(6) Persisting with substance use despite clear evidence of overtly harmful consequences (physical or mental)
(7) Continued substance use despite knowledge of having had a persistent or recurrent physical or psychological problem that was likely to have been caused or exacerbated by the substance	

some pressure to adopt. This pressure to experiment with drugs is all the greater in communities where this behaviour has become so accepted and so acceptable that youngsters believe, often erroneously, that the majority of people of their age are taking drugs and that they themselves are in some way odd or different if they do not. For others, the wish to rebel against the norms of a family or community who disapprove of drug taking may be an equally strong driver.

Although adolescence is a time of non-conformity and unconventionality, it is also a time when peer affiliation and acceptance are crucial. Thus an individual may be introduced to drugs by a close friend, perhaps with the intention of sharing an enjoyable or exciting experience, or to defuse anxiety. Later, however, drug taking may become a focus for group activity and identity when the youngster learns to associate drug taking with socialisation. This, coupled with the pharmacological effects of the drug(s), makes the experience pleasurable and worth repeating. Initially, therefore, drug taking primarily reflects social and cultural factors, including the availability of a particular drug, legal sanctions, media emphasis and so on, whereas subsequent patterns of drug use are more closely related to psychobiological and pharmacological factors. Later still, a frank dependence syndrome may develop, with various physiological effects as well as withdrawal symptoms and craving.

Prevalence

It is not easy to establish the prevalence of substance misuse among young people or the different patterns of consumption, because many will refuse to disclose an illegal activity. Measuring the harm caused by drugs, which in adults can be a useful indicator of substance misuse, is less fruitful among the young as they have not usually been using drugs long enough to cause themselves measurable harm. Furthermore, many studies focus on unrepresentative populations, such as those in remand homes. Also, surveys of educational institutions may be similarly unrepresentative if they exclude students who are absent at the time of survey – absent perhaps because of their drug problem! Furthermore, it is important to clarify what is being investigated in any particular study – whether young people have *ever* taken drugs or whether they are *currently* taking them.

Despite such reservations, it appears that almost half of all young people in the UK try an illegal drug by the age of 16 years and that the average age of first drug use is falling. Alcohol consumption by young people is increasing. Despite the licensing laws, about 60% of children aged between 13 and 17 years have bought alcohol in a pub or off-licence and about one-third drink alcohol at least once a week. This occurs mostly in the home and in small amounts, although drinking to intoxication has also increased. Smoking by this age group is another major public health concern, with the prevalence of smoking having increased from 22% to 29% over a 4-year period. Smoking and drinking by this age group is of particular significance because there is a correlation between the use of illegal drugs and the early use of tobacco, alcohol and volatile substances (Health Advisory Service, 1996; Advisory Council on the Misuse of Drugs, 1998; Wechsler *et al*, 1998).

The aggregated results from several local surveys across the UK show that drug experimentation among pupils increased in the late 1980s and early 1990s, to reach a peak in 1995–96 (Balding, 1999). It was also found that, among a sample of 23 928 pupils surveyed in 1992, 6% of those aged 12–13 years had tried illegal drugs or solvents. This figure rose to 11% at the age of 13–14, 19% at 14–15 and 22% at 15–16; prevalence in the last group had increased to 31% when they were interviewed again in 1993 (Balding, 1999). A recent review from this series of studies seems to show a levelling off, if not a drop in the proportion of 14–15-year-olds who have taken drugs (Balding, 2000), which is consistent with the findings of Miller & Plant (2000). This trend was also apparent in another survey, which found that the use of any drug in the previous year by 16–19-year-olds fell from around one-third in 1994 to just over a quarter in 2000 (Ramsey *et al*, 2001). Perhaps not surprisingly, cannabis is the most popular drug (Institute for the Study of Drug Dependence, 1993).

A survey of the use of alcohol and other drugs in schools across Europe revealed that teenagers in Britain are more likely to drink or take illegal drugs than teenagers in other European countries and start drug use at a younger age (Hibbell *et al*, 1999). In addition, British 15–16-year-old schoolchildren reported the highest lifetime cannabis and solvent use for this age group in Europe (European Monitoring Centre for Drugs and Drug Addiction, 1999). In the most recent report from the United States, drug use among 8th, 10th and 12th graders remains stable; it is reported that more than 50% of high-school seniors experimented with illegal drugs at least once before graduation; during the month prior to the survey, 25% of seniors used illegal drugs and 32% reported being drunk at least once (Office of National Drug Control Policy, 2002). The results from the US National Household Survey on drug misuse revealed that adults who first used cannabis at the age of 14 or younger were five times more likely to be classified as drug dependent or a drug misuser than adults who first used cannabis at age 18 or older (Office of National Drug Control Policy, 2002).

The increasing scale of substance misuse is illustrated by the Regional Drugs Misuse Database report (Sondhi *et al*, 1999), which found that in London the number of drug users under 20 had increased by 35% between 1995 and 1998. In England during the six-month period ending 31 March 2001, about half of those presenting to services with problem drug misuse were in their twenties and about one in seven (13%) were aged under 20 years (Department of Health, 2002).

Risk factors and protective factors

Even with a compassionate, intuitive understanding of the broad underlying reasons for adolescent drug misuse, it is not known why some young people take drugs and experiment with them while others do not, or why some continue to take drugs and become dependent upon them while others cease drug taking before this stage is reached. However, 'risk' factors and 'protective' factors have been identified that throw some light on the different vulnerabilities of young people at different stages of their life.

For example, in early childhood, the development of attachment between child and parents may be impaired, affecting the child in later life and, even at a very early stage in development, early temperamental characteristics of the individual, such as high levels of activity and impulsivity, may be predictive of later problematic behaviour. The latter includes disorders such as attention-deficit hyperactivity and conduct disorder, or behaviours (e.g. aggression) that are themselves insufficient for a diagnosis but are nonetheless troubling. A history of these early characteristics when there is a later, school-age behavioural disorder suggests a developmental disorder, which may have a genetic basis. One view is that there is immature development of the frontal lobes, leading to an inability to direct behaviour towards the pursuit of conventional goals (e.g. parental or teacher praise). Although maturation does occur, with time, the lag between the affected individual and the peer group often persists well into adolescence and, in a minority, persists into adulthood. In some there may be other developmental delays, perhaps involving language, which further compound the difficulties experienced by the young person. Environmental problems in general, and parenting in particular, often come under close scrutiny when behaviour disorders are diagnosed and it is important to acknowledge that a variety of factors may interact. For example, a 'difficult' child is likely to cause stress to the parents, who, especially if they lack support, may be unable to respond in an optimal fashion, resulting in aspects of an attachment disorder. A 'difficult' child will similarly stress teachers, usually leading to further adult criticism and repeated exclusions from school. This in turn impairs academic achievement and it is easy to see how self-esteem is damaged and how the child may find it difficult to trust any adult.

The later stages of childhood and early adolescence are marked by higher rates of conduct and emotional disorders, often with comorbidity of early depressive disorder, anxiety state and conduct disorder. All of

7

these childhood problems may lead to substance misuse and addictive behaviours in adolescence and early adulthood. Other factors that heighten vulnerability include: family disharmony; parental personality disorder or substance misuse; criminal behaviour in the child's close family; physical violence at home; inadequate adult supervision; and stress at home or at school or elsewhere in the child's immediate environment.

During the phase of late adolescence and young adulthood (up to the age of 25 years), the development of independence from the family and adjustment to various social and environmental demands is crucial, with the young person having to learn to meet the everyday challenges of social relationships, educational attainment and employment. These new experiences and demands may invoke anxiety and other emotional reactions and a susceptibility to maladaptive behaviour. Heightened vulnerability to substance misuse at this stage may be noted among those who are homeless (Sibthorpe *et al*, 1995) or who are 'looked after', those with poor academic achievements, truants and school drop-outs (Crome *et al*, 2000), those with learning difficulties and those with mental health problems.

Peer pressure is another factor of crucial importance at this stage. Adolescents and young people wish to be accepted and to feel 'part of the crowd'. Thus the influence of others with whom they associate is especially powerful, affecting the way in which the individual feels and behaves. If the culture of the group and the influence that it exerts is positive and healthy, its dynamic and associated peer pressure can be helpful and constructive. However, it can exert the opposite effect, and may be hard for individual members to resist, if they know that refusing the demands of the group is likely to be followed by rejection. Learning how to select a peer group, how to behave within that group and how to be influential is important both for the individual and for the development of a healthy culture within the group. The positive influence of acceptance within such a group may be an important factor in preventing substance misuse.

Other 'protective' factors include: a warm, happy family and the presence of an adult(s) outside the immediate family with whom young people can develop a trusting relationship; the development of a special talent; the provision of leisure facilities outside school that encourage the development of a healthy lifestyle; and the presence of good, 'achieving' role models (Smith *et al*, 1995).

 Sociology

New technologies

Young people using the internet are at risk from cyber drug dealers and may be exposed to messages promoting drug use. The potential consequences of these developments are alarming. Young people may be drawn into drug-related crime by misinformation, propaganda or brain-washing on the part of unseen individuals whose aim is to profit from a larger drug-using population. When the approach is 'virtual', the warning signals that might deter a young person in the real world are minimised (Ghodse, 2002).

Consequences of substance misuse

For those who do succumb to substance misuse, the consequences can be complex and grave. They include accidental injury, perhaps when driving, or at work, or by being involved in violence, and even death, for example by drowning, burning or fatal falls. There is also a range of less dramatic health problems related to substance misuse – often related to infection (e.g. abscesses, hepatitis, HIV) – which in turn may reflect the mode of drug administration. In addition, there may be mental health problems (e.g. depression) as a consequence of misusing psychoactive substances. Family problems are common, as parents and relatives find it increasingly difficult to cope with a child who persists with substance misuse, and this may culminate in homelessness if the young person is forced to leave the family home or chooses to do so. The need to obtain funds to purchase substances for misuse often leads to criminal behaviour and legal problems, and school exclusion is common.

The serious consequences of substance misuse are particularly poignant when young people are involved and the study of the relationship between illicit drug use and fatalities is therefore con-sidered a priority (Health Advisory Service, 1996). Although it is difficult to determine the precise risk of premature death among addicts, it has been estimated that, overall, teenage addicts (aged 15–19 years) are about 16 times more likely to die than teenagers in the same age group in the general population of England and Wales. Excess mortality is twice as high in females (standardised mortality ratio = 26.5) than in males (standardised mortality ratio = 12.7). Suicide is a factor in this high death rate and it is believed that about one-third of adolescent suicide is associated with intoxication at the time of death (Williams & Morgan, 1994). One cause of a recent increase in youth suicide may be the association with drug and substance misuse (Shaffer *et al*, 1996; Zeitlin, 1999).

Prevention and treatment

None of the consequences outlined above is unique to young substance misusers, but they are all the more disturbing because of their age and because of the justified anxiety that young people may pay too high a price for their youthful misjudgement. Investment in preventing substance misuse and in helping those young people who have already succumbed therefore seems particularly worthwhile. In relation to a reduction in drink-driving, for example, preventive activities could involve a re-examination of societal norms, parental attitudes to drinking and driving, the minimum age for purchasing alcohol, restrictions on advertising, and educational and training programmes for bar staff (Escobedo *et al*, 1995). Family support and life-skills training may also be relevant and successful programmes for school excludees led by those who have previously experimented with drugs have been found to enhance protective factors, encourage pro-social development, improve school performance and decrease drug use (Eggert *et al*, 1994; Kumpfer *et al*, 1996).

It is perhaps common sense that there is greater opportunity for effecting change at the beginning of a potentially damaging drug-taking career rather than later, and, indeed, it has been shown that the earlier an intervention is made, the more likely will be a positive outcome. These early interventions should consist of a general risk-focused approach to help reduce drug use and improve general areas of functioning (Hawkins *et al*, 1992), although there is no evidence that any particular intervention is superior to another (Wagner *et al*, 1999).

Full assessment is, of course, essential and the interventions should address the developmental needs of the child and should be tailored to the individual (Wagner *et al*, 1999). Specifically, the service should be able to track young people over many years so that they do not become 'lost' within the services or allowed to drop out of treatment. To this end, a care pathway of effective and relevant interventions should be devised and it is likely that this will involve a package of care that addresses all aspects of a young person's life, not solely drug use (Green, 1999). In this context it is important to recognise that family-based interventions may be particularly relevant for this age group and that young people may feel alienated in treatment settings dominated by older people, where their own very specific needs cannot be appropriately handled.

A number of issues warrant particular attention when young substance misusers are treated. For example, there are ethical issues about prescribing dependence-producing drugs, especially when their efficacy is not proven in this age group and when their long-term effects are not known. Closely linked to such considerations is the question of whether the goal of treatment is abstinence or harm reduction. If a harm-reduction approach is adopted, this should seek not only to reduce the consequences of drug taking but also to improve other areas of functioning, such as psychiatric and behavioural disorders, school, work, family, criminal behaviour and quality of life generally. However, many feel that abstinence should be the primary goal for all youngsters and that controlled use should not be explicitly acknowledged as a goal, at least initially. As a general principle, packages of care that address all aspects of the young person's life are more likely to be effective than those that focus solely on the substances of misuse, and, given the problems that are often associated with substance misuse, it is not surprising that there is increasing interest in interventions that involve the family as a whole.

There are a number of barriers to treatment for young people. For example, young people who misuse drugs are excluded from services in a variety of different ways. School excludees are not only outside the education system but by their very exclusion are more at risk of further drug taking than if they remained at school. Indeed, by being excluded, their drugs problem may remain unidentified. They are likely to have difficulties such as relationship problems, low self-confidence, an underlying mental health problem as well as financial problems resulting from a need to obtain drugs in whatever way they can (Gilvarry, 1998). Homeless people with drugs problems are particularly difficult to engage and retain in treatment (Kazdin, 1997) and outreach and street-based services should be provided to address the needs of this group.

Dual diagnosis presents another barrier to treatment because psychiatric wards tend to discourage admission of patients with 'drug problems', while many drug services react in a similar way to drug users presenting with a mental health problem. The problems of treating those with a dual diagnosis are all too evident and their exclusion from treatment services can lead to further problems. The young person with these problems has an even smaller repertoire of services to attend (Shaffer *et al*, 1996).

Finally, there are a number of legal issues relating to consent to treatment for young people that are particularly pertinent to the treatment of young substance misusers, especially those who are alienated from their families. In England and Wales, minors aged 16 and 17 can consent to any surgical, medical or dental treatment and the consent of a parent or guardian is not a legal requirement (Department of Health, 1999). While children under 16 cannot generally give consent to treatment, if it is felt that the child has sufficient knowledge and intelligence, then he or she may do so. This is known as 'Gillick competent' (Department of Health, 1999; Standing Conference on Drug Abuse, 1999).

Social services have a responsibility for children up to the age of 16, and if they are already in care, up to the age of 18. The Children Act 1989 enables local authorities to continue to have responsibility up to the age of 21 with regard to accommodation and clothing and for the provision of 'assistance, advice and befriending' (Health Advisory Service, 1996).

Outcome

As always, it is difficult to evaluate the impact of particular inter-ventions, but because the main cause of concern with young people is in areas of personal development (Crome, 1999), it is clear that any measurements of 'improvement' should centre on aspects of psychiatric comorbidity, physical and sexual abuse, criminal activity, prostitution, homelessness, truancy, employment, family functioning and social competencies. Therefore, at the point of assessment, measurements will need to be taken which can then be evaluated after any 'treatment', to determine its effectiveness. Such measurements should include degree of dependence, and problems in relation to physical and psychological health, relationships, legal matters, schooling, and vocational, recreational and housing issues.

Conclusion

Whatever the attitude of individuals and governments to substance misuse by adults, the problem of substance misuse by children is alarming to all. It can and does involve drugs that are controlled under the international conventions, but children are particularly likely to use cheaper substances, such as tobacco, alcohol and solvents, that are not controlled but which may be equally harmful in this age group. Whatever the substance, there is an intuitive acknowledgement that children's immature physiology and, specifically, their developing nervous system and brain may be particularly vulnerable to the effects of drugs. This is compounded by the fear that harmful effects that appear to be transient in adults may cause permanent damage in children, perhaps by harming their mental and physical growth. Children can also be damaged by their involvement in drug production and trafficking, which may be associated with other forms of child exploitation and sexual exploitation in the 'underworld' that harbours all of these activities.

Despite these dangers and fears, there is a rising rate of substance misuse by children and young people worldwide, which can only be tackled with a greater understanding of the nature of the problem and the context in which it arises. For example, strategies to combat substance misuse by children are likely to be different where drugs are a significant part of the country's economy and where drug consumption by the community as a whole is the problem.

Notwithstanding such differences, social, health and educational measures are universally important, while the punitive approaches to substance misuse and drug trafficking that are adopted in many countries seem especially inappropriate for children and young people.

In industrialised countries in particular, as well as in developing countries, popular culture has a profound influence on many young people and it is therefore very important that pop stars and sports idols, who are role models for huge numbers of young people, should not promote or condone substance misuse. The mass media must also act responsibly, conveying consistent and balanced messages, and coherent drug education programmes are required that neither glamorise nor are unnecessarily or unbelievably alarmist. Health services, too, need to be sensitive to the needs of youthful substance misusers and provide age-appropriate responses. Currently, young substance misusers may be excluded from adult services on grounds of age, while paediatric services are often rudimentary.

Despite universal alarm about the rising tide of youthful substance misuse and apparently universal acceptance (enshrined in Article 33 of the Convention on the Rights of the Child) of the need to protect children from substance misuse, this is clearly more difficult to implement in societies where substance misuse by adults is tolerated and where individual rights to use any and all drugs are considered of paramount importance. The need for all professionals in the field to be well educated about the problem and to be responsive to the most vulnerable members of society has never been greater.

References

Advisory Council on the Misuse of Drugs (1998) *Drug Misuse and the Environment*. London: The Stationery Office.

American Psychiatric Association (1994) *Diagnostic and Statistical Manual of Mental Disorders* (4th edn) (DSM–IV). Washington, DC: American Psychiatric Association.

Balding, J. W. (1999) *Young People in 1998 – With a Look Back As Far As 1983*. Exeter: Schools Health Education.

— (2000) *Young People and Illegal Drugs into 2000*. Exeter: Schools Health Education.

Cabinet Office (1998) *Tackling Drugs to Build a Better Britain: The Government's 10-Year Strategy for Tackling Drug Misuse*. London: The Stationery Office.

Crome, I. B. (1999) Treatment interventions – looking towards the millennium. *Drug and Alcohol Dependence*, **55**, 247–263.

— , Christian, J. & Green, C. (2000) The development of a unique designated community drug service for adolescents: policy, prevention and education implications. *Drugs: Education, Prevention and Policy*, **7**, 87–108.

Department of Health (1999) *Drug Misuse and Dependence – Guidelines on Clinical Management*. London: The Stationery Office.

— (2002) *Statistics from the Regional Drug Misuse Databases for 6 Months Ending March 2001*. Department of Health Statistical Bulletin, no. 7. London: Department of Health.

Eggert, L. L., Thompson, E. A., Herting, J., *et al* (1994) Preventing adolescent drug abuse and high school drop out through intensive school based social network development programme. *American Journal of Health Promotion*, **8**, 202–215.

Escobedo, L., Chorba, T. & Waxwieler, R. (1995) Patterns of alcohol use and the risk of drinking and driving amongst U.S. high school students. *American Journal of Public Health*, **85**, 976–978.

European Monitoring Centre for Drugs and Drug Addiction (EMCDDA) (1999) *Annual Report on the State of Drug Problems in the European Union.* http://www.emcdda.org/infopoint/publications/annrep.shtml

Ghodse, A. H. (2002) *Report of International Narcotics Control Board 2001.* Vienna: United Nations Publications.

Gilvarry, E. (1998) Young drug users: early intervention. *Drugs: Education, Prevention and Policy,* **5,** 281–293.

Green, C. (1999) Dependent substance misuse in adolescence: a picture beginning to emerge? *Journal of Substance Use,* **4,** 178–183.

Hawkins, J. D., Catalano, R. & Miller, J. (1992) Risk and protective factors for alcohol and other drug problems in adolescence and early adulthood: implications for substance abuse prevention. *Psychological Bulletin,* **112,** 64–105.

Health Advisory Service (1996) *Children and Young People: Substance Misuse Services: The Substance of Young Needs.* London: HMSO.

Hibbell, B., Anderson, B., Bjamason, T., et al (1999) *Alcohol and Other Drug Use Among Students in 30 European Countries – The 1999 ESPAD Report.* Stockholm: Council for Information on Alcohol and Other Drugs, Council of Europe, Pompidou Group.

Institute for the Study of Drug Dependence (1993) *National Audit of Drug Misuse in Britain.* London: Institute for the Study of Drug Dependence.

Kazdin, A. (1997) Practitioner review. Psychosocial treatments for conduct disorder in children. *Journal of Child Psychiatry and Psychology,* **38,** 161–178.

Kumpfer, K. L., Molgaard, V. & Spoth, R. (1996) The 'Strengthening Families Programme' for the prevention of delinquency and drug use. In *Preventing Childhood Disorders, Substance Misuse and Delinquency* (eds R. Peters & R. McMahon), pp. 241–267. Thousand Oaks, CA: Sage.

Miller, P. & Plant, M. (2000) Drug use has declined among teenagers in the United Kingdom. *British Medical Journal,* **320,** 1536–1537.

Office of National Drug Control Policy (2002) *National Drug Control Strategy.* Washington, DC: White House.

Ramsey, M., Baker, P., Goulden, G., et al (2001) *Drug Misuse Declared in 2000: Results from the British Crime Survey.* London: Home Office.

Shaffer, D., Gould, M., Fisher, P., et al (1996) Psychiatric diagnosis in child and adolescent suicides. *Archives of General Psychiatry,* **53,** 339–348.

Sibthorpe, B., Drinkwater, J., Gardner, K., et al (1995) Drug use, binge drinking and attempted suicide among homeless and potentially homeless youth. *Australia and New Zealand Journal of Psychiatry,* **29,** 248–256.

Smith, C., Lizotte, A., Thomberry, T., et al (1995) Resilient youth: identifying factors that prevent high-risk youth from engaging in serious delinquency and drug use. In *Delinquency and Disrepute in the Life Course* (Current Perspectives on Aging and the Life Cycle Series, no. 4) (ed. J. Hagan), pp. 217–247. Greenwich, CT: JAI Press.

Sondhi, A., Hickman, M., Madden, P., et al (1999) *Annual Report. Data Presented from 1992–1998.* London: Thames Drug Misuse Database.

Standing Conference on Drug Abuse (1999) *Policy Guidelines for Working with Young Drug Users.* London: Standing Conference on Drug Abuse.

Wagner, E., Brown, S., Monti, P., et al (1999) Innovations in substance abuse intervention. *Alcoholism Clinical and Experimental Research,* **23,** 236–249.

Wechsler, H., Rogotti, N., Gledhill-Hoyt, J., et al (1998) Increased levels of cigarette use among college students: a cause of concern. *Journal of the American Medical Association,* **280,** 1673–1676.

Williams, R. & Morgan, H. (1994) *Suicide Prevention – The Challenge Confronted.* London: NHS Health Advisory Service, HMSO.

World Health Organization (1992) *International Classification of Diseases 10 (ICD–10).* Geneva: WHO.

Zeitlin, H. (1999) Psychiatric co-morbidity with substance misuse: children and teenagers. *Drug and Alcohol Dependence,* **55,** 225–234.

CHAPTER 2

Prevention programmes

Ilana B. Crome and Paul McArdle

Key points

- Prevention efforts for adolescents may be providing 'too little too late'.
- There is growing evidence that adequately implemented interventions in childhood are cost-effective ways of reducing substance misuse.
- The valuable components of prevention programmes – largely US-based – are beginning to emerge.
- These include enhancement of parenting or family functioning, booster sessions over two years, interactive teacher–pupil sessions and group social-competence interventions.
- Peer education, didactic teaching and media campaigns lack evidence of efficacy.
- While most prevention programmes are designed to reduce risk factors, it is recognised that enhancement of protective factors is important.
- The role of health care professionals in these developments deserves greater attention, since an understanding of the psychological mechanisms inherent in the initiation and maintenance of substance use and misuse is key to reversing these processes.
- There is a need for implementation and evaluation of long-term prospective UK-based prevention interventions.

Why prevention?

As described in Chapters 1 and 3, surveys have repeatedly demonstrated that the prevalence of substance use, and the range of substances taken by young people, has increased in the past decade. There is little evidence of reduction. It is thus proper to examine the prevention activities that do and do not appear to affect this relentless rise. Types of prevention, specific interventions, and principles of effective prevention are described in this chapter.

What is prevention? Levels, focus and types of prevention

The overall objective of prevention activities is to delay onset of use, to delay progression from lower to higher frequency or quantity of use, or to decrease use. By and large, prevention activities for young people are mainly aimed at alcohol, tobacco and illicit drugs, primarily cannabis. Since regular consumption – usually defined as once a month or once a week – applies to less than 10% of the population, prevention is largely geared towards young people without dependence or withdrawal problems.

Programmes can be conceptualised as focusing on different goals in terms of substance, extent of use, and level of prevention activity (primary or secondary). They can also be categorised in terms of the populations (universal or targeted) at which the activities are directed, and in terms of the different components of the programmes. Although the goal of primary prevention is either to prevent the initiation into or to delay the onset of substance use, prevention of initiation may be an unrealistic objective. Since secondary prevention relates to reducing the level of misuse (i.e. harm reduction or abstinence), it necessarily includes a more complex range of objectives, which match and reflect the varying degrees of substance use or use of different substances. In addition, some prevention strategies aspire to impact indirectly upon the multiple pathways leading to the use and misuse of substances and therefore involve the risk factors that influence childhood and adolescent health and development. Thus, several prevention strategies have emerged.

Two major categories have been described: the 'universal' and the 'targeted' approaches. The universal programmes are available to all children and young people. This approach often focuses on raising awareness and drugs education. One advantage is that there is no 'labelling' or stigmatisation. A disadvantage is that it may be of greatest benefit to those at lowest risk and any significant effect may be difficult to detect. Hence, policy makers may not find this type of programme attractive. By contrast, targeted prevention is for those considered to be at increased risk by virtue of particular characteristics. Prevention targeted on 'external' factors such as social deprivation has been termed 'selective'. Selective prevention may also be aimed at high-risk groups such as school excludees, children with behavioural difficulties and offenders. This approach potentially offers early intervention with multi-disciplinary teams and more efficient use of costly resources.

There are also 'indicated' target interventions, which are directed to 'internal' features such as psychological distress (Offord, 1996).

There follow examples from the literature that illustrate the nature of and types of problems relating to prevention strategies, including evaluation of effectiveness. Depending on the information available, we emphasise features such as research design and methodology. An assessment of a prevention programme will indicate whether the findings provide an adequate evidence base on which to plan and implement policy. It is then critical to question whether the most effective approaches can be practically applied to large groups. Such practicalities relate to the numbers of potential subjects, and the availability, within a reasonable time span, of trained workers in the field. It should be noted that the literature emphasises the 'here and now' nature of the research and the absence of long-term programmes. Furthermore, the interaction of individuals with the wider environment is dynamic, and this changeability should inform the formulation and implementation of strategies.

Universal prevention

Universal prevention encompasses school-based projects as well as those aimed at the general population, including media campaigns. While these are, in general, the key categories, there is very considerable overlap and integration between them. This gives support to the contention that both the problems of substance misuse and the strategies for prevention arise out of factors in the wider community. The factors are subsumed within the school and the structure and dynamics of the family, as well as the individuals at the centre of either potential or existing substance misuse problems. Prevention activity begins in the home, the school playground and the neighbourhood environment.

In most of the studies outlined, programmes concentrate on one substance, primarily cannabis, tobacco or alcohol. However, because of the current 'pick and mix' culture of the young people who misuse substances, the separation of individual substances is now considered to be irrelevant.

Two smoking-prevention studies were reported before the rise of substance misuse in adolescents became apparent. The 1979 Waterloo School Smoking Prevention Trial (Flay et al, 1989) used social influence to raise awareness in 6th grade students. By the 12th grade, programme effects were no longer evident. In the North Karelia Youth Project (Vartiainen et al, 1990), project leaders were used to enhance refusal skills for smoking. After a 15-year follow-up the authors concluded that the intervention delayed smoking uptake but did not prevent it

(Vartiainen *et al*, 1998). The Minnesota Smoking Project (Murray *et al*, 1992) implemented three large-scale school-based projects. Only one, which involved community initiatives, had an influence.

The Alcohol Misuse Prevention Study (AMPS) (Shope *et al*, 1994) focused on reduction by social resistance skills in a high-risk student group. The Western Australian Schools Health and Harm Reduction Project (SHARP) aimed to reduce harm rather than to prevent and delay use. Dealing with high-risk drinking situations was the focus, and positive effects were found.

Multi-component activities

Media campaigns are central to the attempt to mobilise community influences. Pentz *et al* (1989*a*,*b*) reported a randomised trial of school, parent and community multi-component prevention activities; the study employed non-intervention school controls. The programme was based on the selection of appropriate techniques in which teachers and parents were given training in order to inform and assist children in relation to prevention of substance misuse. The school training comprised ten sessions in which role-playing, group discussion and peer facilitation were covered. Teachers received a three-day workshop on 'theory ... and demonstration and practice of sessions'. Parents were involved in six seminars on 'parent–child communication and prevention support skills'. This was combined with a media campaign, which included brief news of the training and implementation of the programme, interviews with project staff and a televised press conference. The authors reported that this Midwestern Prevention Project was associated with a 30% reduction in monthly cigarette use and a 15% reduction in cannabis use over a two-year follow-up compared with controls. With an intervention of such organisational complexity, it is difficult to isolate which components were effective and which, if any, were redundant. Furthermore, although media campaigns constitute the most visible universal interventions, their impact alone is unclear. It should be noted that there was no comment on comparison with controls.

Similarly, Project STAR (Students Taught Awareness and Resistance) (Chou *et al*, 1998) was a two-year multi-component prevention programme involving the media, the community, health policy, the school and the family, together with booster sessions. A follow-up at 18–24 months demonstrated about 25% less use of cannabis, alcohol and tobacco.

Both studies reported use reduction, but not the primary prevention goal, namely that of prevention of onset and initiation into substance use.

School-based prevention

One of the advantages of school-based prevention is ready access to a population at the beginning of and throughout the study period. At its simplest, school-based universal prevention consists of the dissemination of accurate information, rather than an emphasis on scare tactics. In fact, a responsible media role could be helpful, especially if combined with interactive teaching styles (Kumpfer, 1998). In addition to the Pentz and Chou studies, both school-based, those following extend the range and type of school-based approaches.

Drug Abuse Resistance Education (DARE) is a widely adopted programme in the United States. It is curriculum based and includes resistance and personal skills training. Developed by the Los Angeles Police Department, it relied on police officers as 'experts' who gave lectures, held question-and-answer sessions, and facilitated group discussions. This programme has yielded inconsistent results, as meta-analysis of data pooled from a number of evaluations failed to show any effect on substance use (Ennett *et al*, 1994). The data included meta-analysis of both interactive and didactic school-based programmes. When these were analysed separately, interactive techniques yielded a small effect on drug use, whereas the substantial reliance on didactic components, when the young people were not actively engaged in the process, proved to be ineffective. Despite these outcomes, Bauman & Phongsavan (1999) report that 'this program [is] favoured by most schools', underlining the difficulties of translating research findings into practice.

Project ALERT utilised social resistance skills, including psycho-drama, role-play in small-group discussions, and question and answer sessions to increase motivation not to use 'gateway drugs' – cigarettes, alcohol and cannabis (Ellickson *et al*, 1993). Bell *et al* (1993) highlighted the 'here and now' consequences (e.g. 'ashtray breath', losing control), the potential impact on relationships and daily life, and the source of subtle pressure to use such substances. These training exposures took place during eight weekly sessions in year 7 (age 11 years). These were followed by three booster sessions in year 8.

A randomised controlled trial of Project ALERT compared 15 inter-vention and 15 non-intervention schools. Full data were available on 60% of the baseline sample of 6527 participants (Ellickson & Bell, 1990). The intervention was initially associated with reduced cigarette smoking and cannabis use. However, in a longer-term follow-up, Bell *et al* (1993) found no difference in cannabis use between experimental and control groups. Ellickson *et al* (1993) suggested that booster sessions through adolescence might be helpful in prolonging the demonstrated early effect (Ellickson & Bell, 1990). Hence, while Project ALERT demonstrated early effects there were no long-term effects of the two-year programme.

The Life Skills Training programme (Botvin *et al*, 1995; Botvin, 1996) adopted personal and social skills to prevent tobacco, alcohol and marijuana use among students. This comprised a three-year programme, including booster sessions, during 15 school classroom periods. The teacher-led sessions were designed to enhance resistance. Evaluation demonstrated substantially lower levels of smoking and drinking and significantly less use of illicit drugs. Furthermore, these gains were evident after long-term follow-up.

Contrasting Life Skills Training and Project ALERT, it would appear that the former had long-term effects, while those of the latter were short term. This difference may, in part, be due to the extensive 'booster' sessions in subsequent years embedded in the Life Skills Training. It is important to note that the project was tuned to enhance capacities and challenges that adolescents naturally face in their development. These factors were in addition to those aimed directly at substance use.

There are also other innovative examples of school-based prevention. Life Education Centres (LECs) target young children (Hawthorne *et al*, 1995). This approach uses mobile classrooms and eclectic techniques as intervention aids. However, the effectiveness of these approaches has yet to be established. Another, the Illiwara Drug Education Project, includes teaching, group work and peer and parental influence at primary school level. The reported result was that, although fewer children tried nicotine and cannabis, there was no change in alcohol use (Wragg, 1990).

More recently, Spoth and colleagues (Kumpfer *et al*, 1996; Spoth *et al*, 1999) evaluated two school-based prevention projects aimed at improving parent–child relationships: Preparing for Drug-Free Years (PDFY) and the Iowa Strengthening Families Program (ISFP). These were presented as being theoretically distinct. The ISFP was based on a 'bio-psycho-social model' and the PDFY on a 'social development model'. However, it is clear that the components overlap. Preparation for PDFY constituted five two-hour sessions over five weeks. It was mainly with parents and was geared at reducing conflict and increasing 'child involvement in family tasks'. The ISFP was longer, more intensive and more interactive than the PDFY. The ISFP involved seven sessions over seven weeks with groups of ten families. The whole family was involved each week, in addition to separate parent and child sessions. It aimed to enhance the quality of parent–child interactions. Approximately half of those invited agreed to participate, 83% of whom began the programme and approximately 65% completed the programme and follow-up.

As part of the evaluation, the research design included a control condition, in which families received leaflets concerning adolescent development. The authors reported that, compared with the controls, both conditions were effective in preventing progress from non-use to use, the maximal effect being apparent from the 1–2-year follow-up period. There was no significant difference between conditions. Inspection of the data suggested that the differences were located in the transition from no-use or alcohol-only to the next stage (i.e. either tobacco or alcohol use or 'advanced use'). Approximately 30 children of the 193 participants who might have been expected to progress to a more 'advanced' rate of substance use did not do so.

The findings suggest that interactive group programmes that aim to reduce family conflict, promote family integration and have an educational component are effective. The PDFY was less costly, requiring two-person rather than three-person intervention teams, and with the emphasis on parental rather than whole-family involvement. The participants came largely from two-parent, semi-rural or rural families, which raises the question of feasibility in an urban setting. For the UK, there may need to be a further question concerning the social, community and value system differences, compared with the US samples. But the translation of research to practice gives a worthwhile basis for consideration – irrespective of the contextual specifics of the American experience.

General-population-based prevention

As was to be anticipated, many of the issues relating to the general population have emerged in the coverage of the media, the communities, the schools and the family. This section therefore concludes by reporting a novel approach involving the family. It will have become evident that all programmes that involve a large variety of groupings will be costly. Another problem has been that family programmes directed towards general populations typically attract only a minority of eligible families. In an innovative family intervention, Bauman *et al* (2001) randomised families to a leaflet or a telephone interview intervention. The aim of the study was to engage parents and their children in discussion of substance use at an age when decisions about use and non-use are commonly made. Of those eligible (families with a parent and a young adolescent) approximately a third took part, and then were followed up on two occasions over two years using telephone interviews. The intervention was aimed at smoking and alcohol use. There was no effect on alcohol use but, compared with controls, intervention participants reported significantly less smoking. However, the authors were unable to identify how the intervention influenced smoking – whether through family changes or changes in the cognitions of the young person (Ennett *et al*, 2001).

Targeted prevention

In contrast to universal interventions, targeted interventions require the identification of specific groups who require prevention attention. There is the need therefore to screen for high-risk children or young people at increased risk of substance use. There is an inherent problem in this process, since it may lead to the identification of false positives, that is those thought to be at risk but who are not. This, in turn, raises the issue of stigmatisation in an already vulnerable group. Paradoxically, the majority of those found ultimately to have the unwanted outcome may not have been identified by the screening. Nevertheless, despite this, the process does not 'waste' resources on low-risk young people, since targeted interventions are, potentially at least, efficient (Offord, 1996). Furthermore, since at-risk individuals are more likely to engage in more severe substance misuse, successful prevention may assure substantial gains for the wider society and for the individuals themselves.

Selective targeted prevention

In a selective targeted programme (Hawkins *et al*, 1999) pupils attending school in a high-crime area were identified for inclusion. The design included a two-year intervention, a six-year follow-up, and a non-intervention control, but did not include randomisation. The school-based intervention comprised parenting classes, social competence training for the children and teacher training in cognitive–behavioural methods. There was also extensive use of the equivalent of booster sessions. At the six-year follow-up, there was a reduction in a range of antisocial behaviours, including binge drinking, in the intervention group compared with the non-intervention controls. There was evidence of a close relationship between the amount of intervention and outcome. It is also of interest to note that the intervention, despite the lack of randomisation, demonstrated effects on a range of behaviours other than substance use and misuse.

These findings are reinforced by those of Offord (1996), which showed that increasing diversionary activities in a high-crime area was effective in reducing youth antisocial behaviour (which is a risk factor for drug use, although this was not an explicit outcome measure in the Offord study) when compared with an equivalent area without such an intervention programme.

Kumpfer (1998) reported an intervention aimed at increasing the quality of parenting by addressing sensitivity to child cues, effective communication and discipline, and how to play with children. As in the other programmes with similar objectives, there were parallel group work sessions aimed at the social development of children, and family meetings. The intervention took place over 14 weeks and comprised weekly sessions of two to three hours. This programme was both longer and more intensive than the ISFP but in essence the outcomes were similar. Evaluation indicated sustained gains in child behaviour, family relationships and reduced alcohol and tobacco use in older participants.

Of special interest in the UK context, with the presence of a range of ethnic minorities, is the repeated evaluation of the ISFP programme in different groups (urban, rural, African-American and Hispanic) and the evidence of reduced adolescent drug use on longer-term follow-up (Spoth et al, 1999). But underpinning the successful outcomes are a high level of organisation, incentives for families to attend, and adequate staffing. The goals and the resource implications are a very considerable distance from the leaflet and telephone interview approach. Adaptation of this same intervention was applied to at-risk youths identified by self-report of substance use (tobacco, alcohol or drugs).

Chou et al (1998) re-analysed data from the Midwestern Prevention Project and reported that, among those identified as users at baseline, the intervention was associated with reduced cigarette, alcohol and cannabis use, relative to controls. For tobacco and cannabis the maximal effect was evident at 6 and 18 months, but it waned thereafter. However, there was substantial attrition. Over a third of the baseline cannabis users were missing from the intervention, as were half of the control group at six-month follow-up. It is possible that those with the highest risk were the most likely to drop out of follow-up. If this is so, then the measured effects related only to those at relatively low risk. Hence the effect on students at highest risk is unknown, and this is a significant flaw in a targeted intervention. This type of intervention requires further evaluation before it can be considered as a model. Since this intervention is the basis for Project STAR, in the process of dissemination by the US National Institute on Drug Abuse (NIDA), it appears that the published data do not justify this widespread usage.

Among selected targeted interventions, nurse home visiting of vulnerable single mothers has demonstrated explicit reduction in adolescent substance use among children who had been visited until two years of age (Olds et al, 1998). With components of home visiting, promotion of good parenting practices and developmental screening, this programme has clear similarities to the current practice of UK health visitors.

The pre-school education of children from vulnerable families was one of the earliest types of evaluated prevention programme. While these evaluations did not set out explicitly to measure drug use as an outcome variable, various important long-term gains were demonstrated. These Head Start programmes, notably those utilising the High Scope curriculum, have indicated sustained reduction of antisocial behaviour, probably through raising IQ in early school years and so subsequently raising motivation and success in education. Consequently, it is very possible that they had an unmeasured effect on reducing drug use (Dierker *et al*, 2001). Other projects, such as peer-led interventions, are described but do not appear to have been systematically evaluated (Kumpfer, 1998).

While there is an awareness and concern surrounding the preschool child in prevention terms, attention to the prenatal exposures of the unborn child have not been a significant component in all prevention programmes. The evidence of serious damage – physical, neurological and intellectual – resulting from parental substance usage points to a very special case of selective targeting of prevention. Even neonates who appear not to be affected still need ongoing monitoring, since the negative consequences frequently present at a later stage in a child's development (Office for Substance Abuse Prevention, 1992).

Indicated targeted prevention

Indicated targeted interventions focus on children whose early emotional and behavioural problems have been identified. These interventions have been implemented by Kolvin *et al* (1981). McArdle *et al* (2002) report the effect of ten sessions of drama group therapy, delivered by teachers trained in drama therapy. Teachers and parents reported sustained reductions in behavioural and emotional problems among 10–13-year-olds. These UK-based interventions are less elaborate than US studies, less reliant on the use of manuals and more dependent on the professional training of the therapists. However, while these interventions are encouraging, there is need for larger-scale evaluations of their impact on substance use. Biederman *et al* (1999) have demonstrated that effective treatment of childhood behavioural disorders reduced the risk of subsequent substance use disorders in adolescence.

Focus on enhancing protection and resilience

The use of substances by young people often reflects a combination of risk factors (Swadi, 1999). Account needs to be taken of a home environment which may be instrumental in the development of problems. Parental substance use and approval of substance use, family disruption, conflict, poor supervision and disciplinary practices, parent–child conflict, and low parental expectations are all linked. Early onset of smoking is associated with positive expectations of substance misuse, later substance misuse, dependence and psychiatric disorder. The later substance use is initiated, the less likely it is that a young person will have problems. Yet age of onset in itself is not necessarily predictive of addictive behaviour. Misuse and changes in intensity and regularity, that is pattern of use, need to be examined. These may be related to contextual factors, including availability, social deprivation, drug-using peers and those involved in criminal activity.

Stress, strain, low self-esteem and mental health problems (e.g. depression, anxiety), predispose to substance use, as do a history of aggression, impulsivity, hyperactivity and sensation seeking. These aspects are significant because they may mask substance misuse or precipitate problems. In addition, low educational expectations, attainment and achievement – as demonstrated by a poor school attendance record – are likely predictors of substance misuse. The pressing question is how to negotiate with this group of disaffected young people.

Parallel with the prevention theme has been that of risk: risk to the person and also, as with the children of substance misusers, a range of future risks. It appears that there has been little attempt to have disaffected young people define their understanding of risk and their perception of the future outcome of their current reactions to preventive measures. Their involvement and participation may be worthwhile additions to prevention strategies and provide an entry into their community and subculture.

Those factors that are protective, and that may mitigate or inhibit the development of substance misuse, may be of great consequence. These include high self-esteem, high socio-economic status, parental disapproval of substance misuse, family cohesion and attachments with close supervision. Religious involvement, leisure activities, educational aspirations, abilities and achievements are also protective. Awareness of such positive environmental, familial, individual, personality and educational antecedents is vital when designing public health prevention programmes and individual treatment plans.

Comprehensive community-based programmes and control policies embedded in the macro environment: what role for health professionals?

The valuable components of prevention programmes are beginning to emerge. There is a realisation that a spectrum of responses is required for individuals, their families and their peers. There is also the recognition that these are embedded in the wider local community, including the school environment, so due sensitivity to cultural, ethnic and racial diversity is required. Thus, community programmes that include media and policy change should be accompanied by school-based and family interventions. Indeed, schools should offer opportunities to reach all children, to identify and target those most at risk, and to introduce timely prevention programmes. While they are designed to reduce risk factors, the enhancement of protective factors is also recognised as part of the picture.

There is currently a consensus that all substances should be covered. The focus should be on both short-term and longer-term consequences. Smaller programmes, with parental involvement, sustainable over the longer term (perhaps with booster sessions) show promise. The importance of interpersonal skills such as refusal, assertiveness, communication and safety, combined with intrapersonal skills such as coping, self-esteem, stress reduction, problem solving and goal setting, is frequently emphasised. Structured interactive and participating activities, such as role-play, constructive feedback and discussions, sometimes generated by students themselves, are consistently empha-sised as being valuable and effective. This may include discussions about values and the moral and ethical issues that colour attitudes (Tobler, 1997). Unfortunately, recent research on the effects of peer support have not been encouraging (Webster *et al*, 2002).

Furthermore, very specific training in a range of skills also needs to be targeted at high-risk groups. Thus, specific knowledge about attitudes to, and skills in, managing resistance to substances are as important as, and should be linked to, classroom (literacy), leisure (entertainment), extracurricular (drama, sports) and community activities (voluntary work), and also to life skills (job preparation).

Current research should continue to add to the knowledge base. Limitations in the implementation of the range of projects discussed have arisen from the problems of recruitment and retention of subjects, the difficulty of ongoing monitoring of programmes, and the need to adjust and adapt elements so as to meet the fundamental objectives of the programmes. The dynamic nature of the problems makes inter-pretation, especially of cross-sectional data or relatively short-term follow-up, more complicated. Without doubt, longitudinal approaches are required, underpinned by the time and resources necessary to mount such studies. In reviewing these multiple research needs, a system of priorities is required. This, in turn, raises the issue of the need for national research strategies, and for the coordination of policy directions, so that effective prevention programmes can be implemented.

At this point, only a handful of interventions – with the major objectives of reduction of substance misuse, promotion of normal development, and prevention of mental disorder among vulnerable young people – are of proven effectiveness. The vast majority of the efforts deployed to reduce substance use have relied on intuition rather than evidence. Perhaps this explains why the 'net sum of interventions has failed to impact on rising trends in substance use during the early 1990s' (Bauman & Phongsavan, 1999). For this reason Best & Witton (2001) have argued that 'research evidence rather than enthusiasm for a current "prevention fashion" should guide commissioners and prac-titioners'. The importance of relying on the evidence is all the more critical since 'well meaning intervention can do harm' (Dishion *et al*, 1999; LeMarquand *et al*, 2001).

As substance misuse in young people is rising inexorably, there is a natural imperative to undertake prevention activities. Yet, the architects of prevention programmes would do well carefully to consider, implement and evaluate these as part of a national substance misuse strategy. The limited resources available should not be wasted on ineffective efforts. As there are no long-term prospective UK-based prevention interventions, there is an inescapable need – complex as it is – for this type of evaluation.

The potential role of health care professionals merits attention as a research topic since the identification of mechanisms of behavioural change is key to successful implementation of prevention projects. The multifaceted nature of their tasks at different levels can further facilitate their impact on the process of behavioural change. By ensuring ongoing advocacy, by training health and other professionals, by educating children and parents, and by determining policy and research enterprise in their positions of leadership, they could have local, regional, national and, at times, international influence.

While there may be an absence of a national prevention policy, there are a range of initiatives which, if implemented, could constitute 'mini-policies' relating to the use of legal substances (Yu & Shacket, 1998). These relate to the financial and economic aspects of consumption as they are reflected in taxation and price control, as well as media advocacy, the educational institutions, workplace policies, and the use of labelling (e.g. low-fat labelling, the reduced sugar content, the minimal fibre requirements in domestic food products) (Edwards *et al*, 1994). Those producing and selling the legal products should be monitored to ensure that legal requirements relating to age are not breached. Examples of public policies include the imposition of age controls or the regulations requiring health warnings on packaging. MacKinnon *et al* (2000) reported that the addition of a health warning to alcohol beverage containers was associated with a small, transient reduction in drinking by 13- but not 15-year-olds. Further, the government should intervene when, through sponsorship, particularly of sporting events, there is covert advertising of those products banned from the media.

Universal prevention is likely to start with 'healthy public policies' (Brundtland, 2001) aimed at promoting stable families, communities and neighbourhoods, and providing curricula for children that promote success. In other words, the 'macro-environment' or the economic, social and physical aspects of a community, influence the development or reduction of substance problems (Shonkoff & Phillips, 2000; Spooner & Hall, 2002). We conclude that: 'Prevention efforts in adolescents are providing too little too late' and 'there is growing evidence that childhood interventions are cost-effective ways to reduce substance misuse and criminality when they are adequately implemented'. Since the cost and consequences to society are potentially incalculable, prevention programmes are of the essence.

References

Bauman, A. & Phongsavan, P. (1999) Epidemiology of substance use in adolescence: prevalence, trends and policy implications. *Drug and Alcohol Dependence*, **55**, 187–207.

Bauman, K., Foshee, V., Ennett S., *et al* (2001) The influence of a family program on adolescent tobacco and alcohol use. *American Journal of Public Health*, **91**, 604–610.

Bell, R., Ellickson, P. & Harrison, E. (1993) Do drug prevention effects persist into high school? How Project ALERT did with ninth graders. *Preventive Medicine*, **22**, 463–483.

Best, D. & Witton, J. (2001) *Consultation Draft Guidelines for Health Authorities and Social Services*. London: Department of Health.

Biederman, J., Wilens, T., Mick, E., *et al* (1999) Pharmacotherapy of attention-deficit/hyperactivity disorder reduces risk for substance use disorder. *Pediatrics*, **104**, e20.

Botvin, G. J. (1996) Substance abuse prevention through life skills training. In *Preventing Childhood Disorders, Substance Abuse, and Delinquency* (eds R. DeV. Peters & R. I. McMahon), pp. 215–241. Thousand Oaks, CA: Sage.

——, Baker, E., Dusenbury, L., *et al* (1995) Long term follow-up results of a randomized pro-drug abuse prevention trial in a white middle class population. *Journal of the American Medical Association*, **273**, 1106–1112.

Brundtland, G. (2001) The People's Health Assembly (letter). *British Medical Journal*, **323**, 109–110.

Chou, C., Montgomery, S., Pentz, M., *et al* (1998) Effects of a community-based prevention program on decreasing drug use in high-risk adolescents. *American Journal of Public Health*, **88**, 944–948.

Dierker, L., Avenoli, S., Merikangas, K., *et al* (2001) Association between psychiatric disorders and the progression of tobacco use behaviours. *Journal of the American Academy of Child and Adolescent Psychiatry*, **40**, 1159–1167.

Dishion, T., McCord, J. & Poulin, F. (1999) When interventions harm: peer groups and harmful behaviour. *American Psychologist*, **54**, 755–764.

Edwards, G., Anderson, P., Babor, T. F., *et al* (1994) *Alcohol and the Public Good*. Oxford: Oxford University Press.

Ellickson, P. & Bell, R. (1990) Drug prevention in junior high: a multi-site longitudinal test. *Science*, **247**, 1299–1305.

——, —— & McGuigan, K. (1993) Preventing adolescent drug use: long term results of a junior high program. *American Journal of Public Health*, **83**, 856–861.

Ennett, S., Tobler, N., Ringwalt, C., *et al* (1994) How effective is drug abuse resistance education? A meta-analysis of Project DARE outcome evaluations. *American Journal of Public Health*, **84**, 1395–1401.

——, Bauman, K., Pemberton, M., *et al* (2001) Mediation in a family-directed program for the prevention of adolescent tobacco and alcohol use. *Preventive Medicine*, **33**, 333–346.

Flay, B. R., Koepke, D., Thomson, S. J., *et al* (1989) Six-year follow up of the first Waterloo School Smoking Prevention Trial. *American Journal of Public Health*, **79**, 1371–1376.

Hawkins, J., Catalano, R., Kosterman, R., *et al* (1999) Preventing adolescent health risk behaviours by strengthening protection during childhood. *Archives of Pediatrics and Adolescent Medicine*, **153**, 226–234.

Hawthorne, G., Garrard, J. & Dunt, D. (1995) Does Life Education's drug education programme have a public health benefit? *Addiction*, **90**, 205–215.

Kolvin, I., Garside, R., Nicol, A., *et al* (1981) *Help Starts Here: The Maladjusted Child in the Ordinary School*. London: Tavistock.

Kumpfer, K. L. (1998) Selective prevention interventions: the Strengthening Families Program. In *Drug Abuse Prevention Through Family Intervention* (eds R. Ashery, E. Robertson & K. L. Kumpfer). NIDA Research Monograph Series, no. 177: DHHS Pub. No. 99–4135. Washington, DC: Department of Health and Human Services.

——, Molgaard, V. & Spoth, R. (1996) The 'Strengthening Families Program' for the prevention of delinquency and drug use. In *Preventing Childhood Disorders, Substance Misuse and Delinquency* (eds R. DeV. Peters & R. I. McMahon), pp. 241–267. Thousand Oaks, CA: Sage.

LeMarquand, D., Tremblay, R. E. & Vitaro, F. (2001) The prevention of conduct disorder: a review of successful and unsuccessful experiments. In *Conduct Disorders in Childhood and Adolescence* (eds J. Hill & B. Maughan), pp. 449–478. Cambridge: Cambridge University Press.

MacKinnon, D., Nohre, L., Pentz, M-A., *et al* (2000) The alcohol warning and adolescents: 5-year effects. *American Journal of Public Health*, **90**, 1589–1594.

McArdle, P., Moseley, D., Quibell, T., *et al* (2002) School-based indicated prevention: a randomised trial of group therapy. *Journal of Child Psychology and Psychiatry*, **43**, 705–712.

Murray, D. M., Perry, C. L., Griffin, G., *et al* (1992) Results from a state wide approach to adolescent tobacco use prevention. *Preventive Medicine*, **21**, 449–472.

Office for Substance Abuse Prevention (1992) *Monograph 8: Preventing Adolescent Drug Use: From Theory to Practice*. Rockville, MD: Office for Substance Abuse Prevention.

Offord, D. (1996) The state of prevention and early intervention. In *Preventing Childhood Disorders, Substance Misuse and Delinquency* (eds R. DeV. Peters & R. I. McMahon), pp. 329–345. Thousand Oaks, CA: Sage.

Olds, D., Henderson, C. & Cole, R. (1998) Long term effects of home visitation on children's criminal and antisocial behaviour: 15 year follow up of a randomised controlled trial. *Journal of the American Medical Association*, **280**, 1238–1244.

Pentz, M-A., Dwyer, J., MacKinnon, D., *et al* (1989a) A multicommunity trial for primary prevention of adolescent drug abuse: effects on drug use prevalence. *Journal of the American Medical Association*, **261**, 3259–3266.

——, MacKinnon, D., Flay, B., *et al* (1989b) Primary prevention of chronic diseases in adolescence: effects of the Midwestern Prevention Project on tobacco use. *American Journal of Epidemiology*, **130**, 713–724.

Shonkoff, J. P. & Phillips, D. A. (eds) (2000) *From Neurons to Neighborhoods: The Science of Early Childhood Development*. Washington, DC: National Academy Press.

Shope, J. T., Kloska, D. D., Dielman, T. E., *et al* (1994) Longitudinal evaluation of an enhanced alcohol misuse prevention study (AMPS) curriculum for grades six–eight. *Journal of School Health*, **64**, 160–166.

Spooner, C. & Hall, W. D. (2002) Editorial. Preventing drug misuse by young people: we need to do more than 'just say no'. *Addiction*, **97**, 478–481.

Spoth, R., Lopez-Reyes, M., Redmond, C., *et al* (1999) Assessing a public health approach to delay onset and progression of adolescent substance use: latent transition and log-linear analyses of longitudinal family preventive intervention outcomes. *Journal of Consulting and Clinical Psychology*, **67**, 619–630.

Swadi, H. (1999) Individual risk factors for adolescent substance use. *Drug and Alcohol Dependence*, **55**, 209–224.

Tobler, N. (1997) Meta-analysis of adolescent drug prevention programs: results of the 1993 meta-analysis. In *Research Monograph Series, 170* (ed. H. Bukoski), publication no. 97–4146. Rockville, MD: National Institute on Drug Abuse.

Vartiainen, E., Fallonen, U., McAlister, A. L., *et al* (1990) Eight year follow up results of an adolescent smoking prevention program: the North Karelia Youth Project. *American Journal of Public Health*, **80**, 78–79.

——, ——, ——, *et al* (1998) Fifteen year follow up results of an adolescent smoking prevention program: the North Karelia Youth Project. *American Journal of Public Health*, **88**, 81–85.

Webster, R. A., Hunter, M. & Keats, J. (2002) Evaluating the effects of a peer support programme on adolescents' knowledge, attitudes and use of alcohol and tobacco. *Drug and Alcohol Review*, **21**, 7–16.

Wragg, J. (1990) The longitudinal evaluation of a primary school drug education programme: did it work? *Drug Education Journal of Australia*, **4**, 33–44.

Yu, J. & Shacket, R. (1998) Long term change in under age drinking and impaired driving after the establishment of drinking laws in New York State. *Alcohol Clinical and Experimental Research*, **22**, 1443–1449.

CHAPTER 3

The epidemiology of substance misuse in young people

Martin Frischer, Paul McArdle and Ilana B. Crome

Key points

- Among people aged 16–24 years in England and Wales, 24% (2.3 million) reported using drugs in the previous year in the 2000 British Crime Survey. Within this group, 533 000 had used class A drugs in the previous year and 275 000 in the past month.
- Teenagers in Britain are more likely to have taken illegal drugs or drink than their counterparts anywhere else in Europe. Furthermore, they appear to start drug use at a younger age.
- The high rate of female binge drinking may be particularly important in terms of its potential contribution not only to teenage pregnancies but also to developmental problems in the foetus.
- Household survey data indicate that the overwhelming majority of people use illicit drugs only for a relatively short time.
- Although some risk factors for young people's drug use have been identified (e.g. not living with both parents), these may be extremely difficult to modify.
- Evidence from new 'outbreaks' of drug use is that they are supply led rather than demand driven and efforts to reduce demand (e.g. via education) are controversial.
- Epidemiological studies alone cannot determine for what reasons, or 'why', and by what mechanisms, or 'how', substance misuse develops.

Introduction: the conceptual framework

Epidemiology is concerned with the pattern of disease occurring in human populations and the factors influencing these patterns (Lilienfeld & Stolley, 1994). Epidemiologists try to determine whether disease prevalence changes over time or over geographical area, and its associations with personal and social characteristics. In recent years,

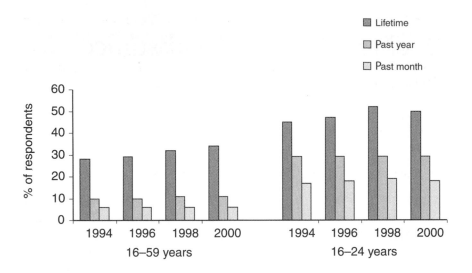

Figure 3.1 British Crime Surveys, 1994–2000: proportion of respondents reporting any illicit drug use (2000 sample, *n* = 13 021).

there has been an explosion of drug misuse epidemiology with regard to methodological developments and substantial research. However, not all commentators accept the concept of 'drug use epidemiology', as it implies that drug use is a disease or is analogous to a disease. There are many alternative viewpoints, for example that drug use is a matter of individual choice (Davies, 1992). In a more sophisticated version of this view, explanations for drug use are seen as dependent on a complex interplay of personal and social factors, including deprivation (Rutter & Smith, 1995). However the issues are conceptualised, substance misuse is a major cause of global morbidity and premature mortality (Harvard School of Public Health, 2002). Suicide, accidents, violence, intoxication and overdose contribute to this picture.

Until the late 1970s, Britain's drug problem was of international interest only because of the insignificance of its size (Ditton & Frischer, 2001). Then, in the early 1980s, there appears to have been a dramatic upsurge, which has continued unabated to the present day. Figure 3.1 shows that in the 2000 British Crime Survey (BCS) (Ramsey *et al*, 2001) 34% of the adult population had used an illicit drug; among people aged 16–24 the figure was 50%. Figure 3.1 also indicates that the vast majority of people do not persist with drug use. This can be estimated by calculating the proportion of lifetime users who have also used in the past month. Monthly continuation rates are 18% and 36% for those aged 16–59 and 16–24, respectively.

Unfortunately, the BCS does not cover alcohol and tobacco use, but Dutch data show that monthly continuation rates are 88% for alcohol, 88% for tobacco, 16% for cannabis, 14% for ecstasy and 10% for heroin (Abraham *et al*, 1998). These simple observations from household surveys raise important epidemiological questions about drug use and its relationship to drug dependence. Most obviously, it is evident that the overwhelming majority of people use drugs for only a relatively short time.

Definition of drug use and drug dependence

Very little of the drug use represented in Figure 3.1 will ever reach the attention of medical, criminal justice or social services. The vast majority of respondents will not regard themselves as being dependent on drugs. The ICD–10 definitions (World Health Organization, 1992) (see Tables 1.1 and 1.2, pp. 3, 4) illustrate the complexity, from both a substantive and a semantic point of view, of the criteria required for a diagnosis of harmful use or dependence. For example, what is meant by compulsion? Is this to be assessed from self-report, or from observation of drug-seeking behaviour? In general, dependence is a condition diagnosed by experienced practitioners. Thus, in order to assess harmful, 'problematic' or dependent drug use, it is necessary to turn to statistics that record people who come into contact with services, although great caution is required. For example, many young people who have a service contact may not be dependent according to the ICD–10 definition.

Epidemiological methodologies

Given the range of drug use, it is important to be clear about what objectives can be met by different epidemiological methodologies. Eleven epidemiological methods are considered by Frischer (1996) in terms of financial resources, statistical expertise and fieldwork. Another dimension relates to whether the drug use is local, national, urban, rural, 'recreational' or 'problematic'.

Household surveys yield information on general trends in the population but are not suitable for assessing, say, the level of problematic heroin use or dependence. School surveys can provide critical information on early experiences of drugs, but may not be able to capture important contextual information such as can be derived from qualitative interviews. Although rarely acknowledged, survey responses are sensitive to the settings in which the questions are asked (Davies, 1992).

Routine sources provide data on drug users who come into contact with medical, criminal justice and social service agencies. These can be useful for providing a cross-sectional snapshot. However, some reporting systems have different definitions and reporting frameworks, which can make trends difficult to evaluate.

Analytic and case control studies are required to move beyond descriptive epidemiology. For example, the link between smoking and cancer would not have been established without detailed analysis of a cohort of British doctors over a long period of time. Unfortunately, these types of longitudinal data are rarely available for drug use, in part because of its illegal status. It is possible to assemble only some pieces of the jigsaw at this point in time.

This chapter addresses five issues:

- What are the current levels of overall use and problematic substance use among young people?
- What are the trends in substance use among this population?
- Do epidemiological studies indicate causal factors for substance use among young people?
- Does epidemiological evaluation of risk suggest preventive measures?
- How do the epidemiological data relate to service provision?

With regard to the epidemiological issues, the chapter confines itself to epidemiological studies and does not consider the voluminous literature on substance use that does not have an epidemiological focus.

Current levels and trends

Substance use among young people in the general population

Figure 3.1 shows levels of drug use among the population aged 16–59 and 16–24 in England and Wales. The 2000 sweep of the BCS (conducted in England and Wales) found that, among people aged 16–24, 24% (2.3 million) reported using drugs in the previous year. Within this group 533 000 used class A drugs in the past year and 275 000 in the past month (Ramsey *et al*, 2001). Use of 'any drug' in the past year by 16–19-year-olds fell from around a third in 1994 to just over a quarter by 2000 (Ramsey *et al*, 2001). Use of class A drugs remained fairly stable for 16–24-year-olds between surveys, with use in the past year increasing slightly from 8% in 1998 to 9% in 2000; use in the past month increased from 3% in 1998 to 5% in 2000. Neither increase was statistically significant.

Data from the 2000 survey included an ethnic booster sample to enable sensitive analyses of the differences in drug use across ethnic groups. In addition to the main sample of 19 411, the booster included interviews with 3874 respondents. The main ethnic groups compared are White, all Black groups, Indian and Pakistani/Bangladeshi. The category of 'all black groups' was referred to in previous BCS reports as 'Afro-Caribbean'. Then and now, this covers 'Black Caribbean', 'Black African' and 'Black other' categories. The new term has been adopted to reflect more appropriately the heterogeneity of this group and to be consistent with the most recent BCS reports on non-drug-related topics. Participation rates for the drugs component of the 2000 BCS were 98% for Whites; 96% for Black people; 92% for Indians, and 81% for Pakistani/Bangladeshis.

In the 2000 BCS, among those aged 16–29 (Table 3.1), nearly half (46%) of all White people reported ever having taken cannabis and nearly a quarter (22%) reported ever having used any class A drug. With the exception of crack, young White people consistently had higher prevalence rates for all the types of lifetime drug use shown. Lifetime use of heroin, cocaine, ecstasy and amphetamine by the Indian ethnic group equated with or exceeded that of young Black people. Pakistani/Bangladeshi lifetime drug use rates remained low in comparison with other ethnic groups.

Approximately 20% of problem crack users presenting for treatment were from Black minority ethnic groups, compared with 50% of crack users assessed by arrest referral workers (London Health Observatory, 2003). It is possible that drug users from Britain's Black communities are more likely to remain unknown to service agencies – reflecting disadvantage in access to health care (Awiah et al, 1990). However, Leitner et al (1993) also noted that, although ethnic respondents in the Drug Use and Drug Prevalence Study were more likely to be of lower socio-economic status, their level of reported drug use did not exceed that of the white population. In summary, there are conflicting views on patterns of drug use among ethnic minorities: some studies report high levels, while others report similar levels to the White population.

Drug misuse largely remains an uncommon or a short-lived activity. While a third of those aged 16–59 have tried illicit substances at some time in their lives, rates of drug use for the past year and past month are much lower, at 11% and 6%, respectively. The vast majority of people in the UK who use drugs, even those in deprived areas, do so infrequently (Ramsey & Partridge, 1999). Cannabis remains the most widely consumed prohibited substance, tried by almost half of 20–24-year-olds. Around half of all drug users restrict themselves simply to cannabis (Ramsey & Partridge, 1999). In the 2000 BCS, 58% of people aged 16–24 who had 'ever' used drugs had continued to use them in the past year and 36% in the past month. Survey data also indicate that, contrary to widespread belief, so-called 'addictive' drugs may not be difficult to give up. Figure 3.2 shows the response of young drug users in 10 European

Table 3.1 Percentage of respondents aged 16–29 years using various drugs in their lifetime, by ethnic group (BCS 2000)

	White	All Black groups	Indian	Pakistani/ Bangladeshi
Cocaine	10	6	7	1
Crack	2	3	2	–
Heroin	2	–	1	–
Amphetamine	**23	6	6	2
Ecstasy	**12	5	7	2
Cannabis	**46	32	21	9
Class A	**22	9	9	3
Any drug	**52	37	25	13

**Significant difference between Whites and all other main ethnic groups at $P < 0.01$.
Data on the Chinese ethnic group are not included due to small numbers in the sample ($n = 50$).
Source: BCS 2000, core and booster samples (weighted data).

cities when asked 'which of the substances they were taking would be the most difficult to give up' (Calafat *et al*, 1999).

In the Nightlife study (Calafat *et al*, 1999) there was also growing evidence that heroin use was increasing among young people from ethnic minority (predominantly South-East Asian) backgrounds. There was particular concern that the exploding Asian youth population could fall into very real difficulties if this trend continues. Those who had some knowledge of drug use patterns in ethnic minority groups felt that stimulants such as amphetamine and ecstasy were unpopular, with only very low levels of use in comparison with drugs such as cannabis and cocaine. It was felt that this trend had a lot to do with the image of these drugs as being 'a White man's drug'.

The British General Household Survey in 1998 (Bridgwood, 2000) confirmed extensive alcohol consumption among young adults (aged 16–24 years). Twelve per cent of young men were drinking between 4 and 8 units of alcohol daily, and 35% were drinking over 8 units daily. In women, 40% were exceeding 3 units daily. Seventeen per cent were drinking between 3 and 6 units a day and 23% were drinking more than 6 units a day.

Another recent report suggests that heavy drinking in young British women gives cause for concern (Plant & Plant, 2001). The highest proportion of women who were high-risk drinkers (>35 units per week) were in the 18–24-year age group, compared with the 35–54-year age group for men (>50 units per week. The implication of these findings is the increasing likelihood that young women will present to services with alcohol-related psychosocial and physical problems.

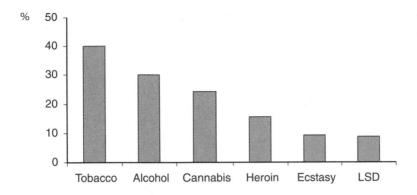

Figure 3.2 The drugs rated as the most difficult to give up (by those who had consumed them in the previous year) (adapted with permission from Calafat *et al*, 1999).

Surveys among people of school age

The proportion of pupils aged 11–15 who used drugs in the past month increased from 7% in 1998 to 9% in 2000 (National Centre for Social Research & the National Foundation for Educational Research, 2001) (Table 3.2). The proportion who had used drugs in the past year increased from 11% to 14% over the same period. In 2000, cannabis was by far the most likely drug to have been used – 12% of pupils aged 11–15 had used cannabis in the past year. Use of cannabis in the past year was slightly higher among boys (13%) than girls (11%). Cannabis use increased sharply with age: 2% of 11-year-olds had used the drug in the past year compared with 28% of 15-year-olds.

The government has expressed particular concern about the use of heroin and cocaine, as these are considered the drugs that cause the greatest harm. In 1999, 1% of 11–15-year-olds had used opiates (heroin or methadone) in the past year, and 4% had used stimulants (a group of substances that includes cocaine and crack as well as ecstasy, amphetamines and poppers). The proportions of pupils using these types of drugs are small and the survey did not detect any differences between 1998 and 2000 (National Centre for Social Research & the National Foundation for Educational Research, 2001). However, among 16–19-year-olds the use of cocaine in the previous year increased from 1% in 1994 to 4% in 2000 (Ramsey *et al*, 2001).

According to the 1998/1999 European School Survey Project on Alcohol and Other Drugs (ESPAD) (Hibbell *et al*, 2000), teenagers in Britain are more likely to have taken illegal drugs or drink than their

Table 3.2 Estimates of drug use among the population aged under 25

Survey	Population age (years)	Category	Estimated no. of drug users
British Crime Survey	16–24	Any illicit drug: lifetime	2 882 200
British Crime Survey	16–24	Any illicit drug: past year	1 671 676
British Crime Survey	16–24	Any illicit drug: past month	1 037 592
British Crime Survey	16–24	Class A: lifetime	1 152 880
British Crime Survey	16–24	Class A: past year	518 796
British Crime Survey	16–24	Class A: past month	288 220
National Centre for Social Research	11–15	Any illicit drug: past year	450 950
National Centre for Social Research	11–15	Any illicit drug: past month	289 665
Multiple Indicator Method	Under 25	Problematic	103 732

All estimates relate to 2000, except the multiple indicator method estimate, which relates to 1996. The population is 2 218 500 aged 11–15 and 5 764 400 aged 16–24.

counterparts anywhere else in Europe. Furthermore, they appear to start drug use at a younger age.

They are also near the top of the league when it comes to smoking cigarettes. The ESPAD study confirmed the extent of nicotine use among young British people. Almost 70% have tried cigarettes and one-quarter of young people have used cigarettes more than 40 times in their lives, which is an indication of regular use. One-third have smoked in the past 30 days: this includes first time and regular use. A new phenomenon in the UK is that girls are in the majority and exceeding boys in nicotine use. Twenty per cent of 13-year-olds are smoking daily and by 15 this has increased to 25%. Not surprisingly, there is a high correlation between lifetime prevalence and the proportion of students in the UK who smoked their first cigarette at 13 years or younger. This is further discussed in Chapter 9.

The first ESPAD survey (Hibbell et al, 1997) reported that, in the UK sample, 20% of 15–16-year-old girls and 24% of boys acknowledged binge drinking (five drinks or more in a row) in the past 30 days. In the 1999 sequel, this had risen to 27% and 33%, respectively. In 1999, 94% admitted to ever having used alcohol, and 47% had used it 40 times or more. The vast majority, 91%, had used alcohol in the past year, and a third had had a drink 20 times or more in the previous 12 months. The proportion reporting drunkenness in the previous year, 69%, was higher than the European average of 52%. Three-quarters had been drunk once, but about 50% had been intoxicated or had binged once in the past 30 days and 25% had been intoxicated or binged three times in the previous month.

The UK has one of the highest rates of lifetime alcohol use, drunkenness, intoxication and binge drinking in Europe. These rates are approximately joint second with Ireland from 30 countries surveyed, somewhat behind Poland. Although the rates were not calculated in an identical fashion, they are comparable to the reported behaviour of US young people (Center on Addiction and Substance Abuse, 2002). Perhaps not surprisingly, the rate of drunkenness (three times or more in the past 30 days) acknowledged by girls had also risen, from 20% to 25%. However, the rate of male drunkenness had remained unchanged, conceivably reflecting tolerance. If this is the case, then it reflects chronic high levels of drinking, with the major risk of a surge of alcohol-related health problems in a decade or two. The high rate of female binge drinking may be particularly important in terms of its potential contribution not only to teenage pregnancies but also to developmental problems in the foetus.

The major limitation of this kind of approach is the fact that many young people who are using substances are not attending school. An alternative approach was pioneered in an Europe-wide study (Calafat *et al*, 1999). The Nightlife survey covered nine European cities (Athens, Berlin, Coimbra, Manchester, Modena, Nice, Palma de Mallorca, Utrecht and Vienna). Information was obtained from a wide range of young people and key informants associated with the nightlife scene. The results indicate that the prevalence of drug use was higher in Manchester than other cities and drug users in Manchester tended to start using drugs at an earlier age than their European counterparts. Informants felt that drug taking among young people was very prevalent and that drugs were generally widely available. The bulk of drug users that they came across were in the 17–25-year age group, but they felt that drugs were taken by a wide range of people, with ages ranging from as young as 9 years right up to 60 years and over. It was also felt that the range of drugs available for people to choose from was getting wider. Although the extent of drug use was felt to be generally very high, informants made a distinction between 'recreational' drug users and 'dependent' or 'chaotic' drug users. 'Recreational' drug users were seen as those individuals who would mostly restrict their use to their spare time and for the most part did not consider their use to be a problem. The more 'dependent' or 'chaotic' drug users were those who were often addicted to and in many cases injecting drugs such as heroin, crack cocaine and amphetamine. These users were considered to be more likely to run into difficulties either with their physical or mental health or with the criminal justice system. They were considered primarily to consist of people who were more socially dislocated and often suffering multiple deprivations – unemployed, marginalised, poorly educated, with poor family and social relationships.

Recently, there has been concern regarding flunitrazepam. This drug is part of the benzodiazepine family of drugs and has been implicated in a number of 'date rape' cases in America. There was growing evidence that this drug may be becoming misused in England. This was a particular concern of the police, who felt that in the wrong hands this drug could be used to force sexual advances on women. However, most key informants in the Nightlife study (Calafat *et al*, 1999) had not heard of anyone who had actually experienced a sexual assault or had been attacked as a result of being 'spiked' with this drug; however, some members had heard of it being misused.

Notified drug 'addicts'

In 1961 the report of the Interdepartmental Committee on Drug Addiction, chaired by Sir Russell Brain, noted that 'on the evidence before us the incidence of addiction to dangerous drugs is very small ... there seems no reason to think that any increase is occurring' (see Lawrie, 1978). The UK addict population was thought to be about 400, mostly elderly people who contracted the habit through medical treatment. There were an estimated 70 doctors and nurses who were addicts and perhaps a dozen non-medical addicts. In 1964 there was a sudden increase in the number of notified addicts (mainly young people) and the committee was reconvened in 1965. Data from the Home Office Addicts Index (HOAI) are shown in Figure 3.3. The HOAI was discontinued after 1997 and replaced by Regional Drug Misuse Databases (RDMDs). Unlike the HOAI, which recorded new and renotified addicts each year, the RDMDs record only new agency contacts and re-attenders after a six-month gap, so it is not possible to provide comparable figures beyond 1997.

Problematic drug use

What is 'problem drug use'? As described in Chapter 1, the current (ICD–10) definition of harmful use and dependence in part consists of 'a cluster of behavioural, cognitive and physiological phenomena that develop after repeated substance use'. In practice, the latter definition is difficult to implement in national prevalence studies, which tend to be based on routine data sources. In contrast, in 1998 a working group of the European Monitoring Centre for Drug Dependence and Abuse (EMCDDA) defined 'problematic drug use' as 'intravenous drug use or long duration/regular use of opiates, cocaine and/or amphetamines. Ecstasy and cannabis are not included' (Kraus *et al*, 1998). This definition does not mention anything about the users' perception of their drug use, but it is easier to apply as an estimate of severity of drug use.

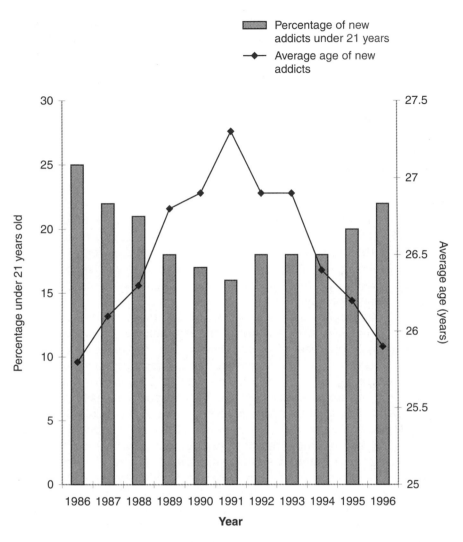

Figure 3.3 Numbers of notified addicts in the UK according to the Home Office Addicts Index (adapted with permission from Ghodse, 2002)

One way of estimating the numbers of 'problematic' users in Britain has been to gather information on people presenting to treatment services. In the 6-month period ending 30 September 2000, 33 093 people were reported to have started drug treatment episodes in England (Department of Health, 2000). The number of drug misusers reported by drug treatment agencies and general practitioners (GPs) in England as presenting for treatment has increased steadily, from 16 810 for the 6-month period ending 30 September 1993 to 33 093 for the 6-month period ending 30 September 2000 (Department of Health, 2000). About one in seven (14%) were under 19 years of age, but the majority (68%) were aged between 20 and 34 years. The age/gender distribution shows that a greater proportion of young women (16%) than young men (11%) were between the ages of 15 and 19 years.

The most reliable method of estimating 'problematic users' is probably the Multiple Indicator Method (MIM). This estimation of the number of problem drug users in the population involves combining information on prevalence that is available only in a few areas (otherwise known as 'anchor points' or the calibration samples) with 'indicators' or 'predictors' of drug use (e.g. criminal justice data). These are available in all areas. Estimates for the UK are shown in Table 3.3. The UK estimate for 1996 was 268 253. If the age breakdowns for known users in 1997/8 are used (Department of Health, 1999), then 112 666 (42%) of the estimated problematic users were aged under 25 years.

Zoccolillo *et al* (1999) examined 'problem use' and reported that approximately 75% of those who had 'ever' misused illicit drugs had done so more than five times. Sutherland & Shepherd (2001) describe a similar phenomenon and suggest that among those youths who admit to any cannabis misuse their use is not experimental but appears to be frequent. Of the 'regular' users identified by Zoccolillo *et al* (1999), 44.7% of boys and 26.9% of girls reported engaging in sport under the influence of alcohol, 33.6% of boys and 25.5% of girls had drunk alcohol in the morning, and 16% and 13%, respectively, had been drunk at school. The corresponding percentages of illicit drug users were 75.2% and 53.3% for use of drugs while engaging in sport, 68.0% and 55.7% for use of drugs in the morning, and 79.1% and 69.4% for 'drugged or high while at school'. In addition, among the drug users, substantial minorities had been intoxicated while driving, had been in fights or had had rows with parents because of illicit drug use. The authors concluded that 'normative drug use ... was use several times a

Table 3.3 UK selected drug indicators and Multiple Indicator Method prevalence estimates per 10 000 population, 1996

UK regions	Indicator 1: convictions	Indicator 2: treatment	Anchor point	Prevalence estimate
Northern and Yorkshire	17.20	14.73		55.7
North Thames	24.61	10.91	61.8	57.3
South West	17.29	9.61		47.3
West Midlands	13.83	8.39	25.5	18.7
North West	20.01	14.28		69.3
Wales	21.55	8.05	29.5	44.5
Great Britain	16.84	11.40		48.8

Simplified and adapted from Frischer (2001). Full model contains five indicators.

week, attending school stoned, playing sports stoned and using drugs in the morning'. The data do not specify concrete impairment such as 'a failure to major role obligations' as required by DSM–IV, so that these findings fall short of 'substance abuse' criteria (American Psychiatric Association, 1994). These data do suggest that 'use' may not be quite the non-malign practice that the deliberately non-judgemental term implies.

The DSM–IV diagnosis of substance use disorder (SUD) relies on the presence of either dependence or abuse (American Psychiatric Association, 1994). As part of a larger epidemiological study, Shaffer et al (1996) estimated the rate of SUD (alcohol or drugs) at 2.0% of a population of 1275 young people aged 9–17 years. Since misuse is more likely to occur in older subjects, this overall rate might be a substantial underestimate of rates in middle or later adolescents. As part of a German study of early developmental stages of psychopathology, Perkonigg et al (1999) examined rates of cannabis dependence by interviewing a representative sample of Munich adolescents aged 14–17. They reported a rate of 2.0% for 'heavy use' ('at least 2–3 times per week'). At follow-up, on average 19.7 months later, the cumulative lifetime incidence was 3.8%. This rate is similar to the 3.8% of Bremen 15- and 16-year-olds reporting poly-drug use (McArdle et al, 2002). Perkonigg et al (1999) reported rates for 'abuse' that were approximately similar: 1.9% at baseline and 2.7% at follow-up. Many of these young people were concurrent users of other drugs and these rates might be a reasonable approximation of rates of illicit drug misuse as a whole. The authors noted that their rates of 'abuse' were lower than the 5.6% obtained from the US National Comorbidity Survey (Anthony et al, 1994). Hence, overall, it appears that rates of diagnosable substance misuse and dependence are likely to be between 2% and 6% of youth populations. To some extent, the variation depends on where the youth lives, and this is likely to relate to availability (Hofler et al, 1999; McArdle et al, 2000). Nevertheless, a degree of perspective is required, as alcohol and nicotine remain the most widely used drugs and may also be the most addictive (see Figure 3.2).

Do epidemiological studies indicate causal factors for substance misuse among young people?

Numerous factors have been reported to be associated with increasing drug misuse: greater individualism and consumerism in the post-war era, weakening of family relationships and lengthening periods of adolescence (Rutter & Smith, 1995). Recent British surveys have found interpersonal and environmental factors to be associated with drug use (Leitner et al, 1993; Ramsey & Percy, 1996). However, these associations explain only a small amount of variability in drug use. It has been observed that:

'with such widespread drug trying ... it is unlikely that the search for "risk factors" in terms of indicators of personality disorder and social malaise will be adequate. Such analyses will link social exclusion with problematic drug use but will have little potency in predicting the scale or range of future problem users in such a large normative population of ordinary youth.' (Aldridge *et al*, 1999).

Even when studies have shown strong associations, it is difficult to separate cause and effect. In the example of smoking and lung cancer it is fairly non-contentious that smoking causes lung cancer and not vice versa. As most drug studies are cross-sectional, the direction of causality is hard to interpret. Recent longitudinal studies from the United States indicate that important risk factors for *later* drug use are age of initiation (Hawkins *et al*, 2000), friends smoking around the time of school leaving (West *et al*, 1999), weaker decision-making skills and negative perceptions of school. These are not risk factors that are easily modifiable. Data from the UK indicate that people in deprived areas report much higher levels of drug use. Does this mean that deprivation is a causal factor? The majority of young people in these areas do not report using drugs, so it is unclear whether deprivation *per se* is the causal factor or whether it has a more complex interaction with other factors.

McArdle *et al* (2002) reported that living with both parents and the quality of the parent–child relationship were associated independently with drug use by young people: in the absence of either the family structure or 'quality' variables, the rate of drug use was 42.3%; if both were present it was 16.6%; and in the presence of either, approximately 32%, suggesting an additive relationship. Hence, the rate of drug use in modern urban communities would remain substantial even in the absence of family risk factors, but short of the 'normalisation' described by Parker *et al* (1998).

Does epidemiological evaluation of risk suggest preventive measures?

In 1992 Jane Griffin wrote that society, faced with the sharpness and complexity of changes in drug use, shows 'a degree of confusion, panic or rush for solutions, in dealing with the problem' (Griffin, 1992). One area in which this is manifest is drug education. The current consensus is that 'evaluations that have attempted to demonstrate results in terms of reducing or preventing drug use have proved inconclusive' (LocateNet, 2001), while Lloyd & Joyce (1999) reported that British studies deal with process issues and 'outcomes ... at barely more than the anecdotal level' (see also Chapter 2). Nevertheless, the government's Anti-Drugs Coordinator reports that 'educating children about the risks associated with drugs can delay or avoid the start of experimentation' (United Kingdom Anti-Drugs Coordinator, 2001). In contrast, Martin Plant (currently Professor at the Alcohol and Health Research Centre, University of the West of England) was quoted as saying that 'anti-drugs campaigns are more likely to encourage young people to experiment with drugs' and 'high profile campaigning may be seductive for politicians, but it is simplistic. Media advertising is simply a waste of money' (Gallacher & Gray, 2002).

The government objective for people under 25 is to reduce the proportion using class A drugs by 25% by 2005 and by 50% by 2008. There are many initiatives to achieve this goal. For example, £7 million was made available from 1998 over four years for work with vulnerable young people in the 26 Health Action Zones (HAZs). This funding has supported a number of intervention projects in some of the most deprived parts of the country. These projects have been targeted at young people at particular risk of developing problems with drug misuse, including young offenders, homeless young people, 'looked after' children, children excluded from school, and children whose parents misuse drugs. An Office of Her Majesty's Chief Inspector of Schools (Ofsted) report (Ofsted, 2000) on drug, alcohol and tobacco education in 1500 schools showed marked improvement since 1997. In 1997, 86% of secondary and 61% of primary schools had drug, alcohol and tobacco education policies; by 1999 that figure had risen to 93% and 75%, respectively. However, as yet, there is no evidence regarding implementation of policies, or on their effects on young people's health.

In addition, the available evidence from new 'outbreaks' of drug use is that they are supply led rather than demand driven. Our own data from a survey of regular drug users in Ayrshire, Scotland (Figure 3.4; further details available from the authors on request) clearly show that the vast majority of young people report using drugs to provide pleasure. Thus, the efficacy of drug prevention initiatives centred on demand reduction by highlighting the risks of drug use, which do not relate to the reasons young people themselves give for taking drugs, must be questioned. As with many other activities that are pleasurable, young people do not worry too much about the long-term consequences, particularly where the impact is not obvious and the evidence is not strong. With regard to problematic use, the minority who use drugs to stop themselves from feeling bad are a more vulnerable group in terms of drug use becoming problematic, and are the group more likely to present to treatment agencies with a comorbid condition or with established substance misuse.

How do the epidemiological data relate to service provision?

The Health Advisory Service reports *Children and Young People Substance Misuse Services: The Substance of Young Needs* (1996, 2001) describe four levels or 'tiers' of service provision, which, taken together, create an infrastructure within which purposeful intervention can occur. The four tiers are:

Tier 1   Generic services with direct access to young people which are able to provide drug education, information and referral of young drug users.

Tier 2   Youth-orientated services, which are able to provide all of Tier 1, plus drug-related prevention and targeted education, advice and general counselling services using a multi-disciplinary approach.

Tier 3   Key professionals, who can provide specialist drug services and other specialist services that work with complex cases requiring multi-disciplinary team-based work.

Tier 4   Very specialised and intensive forms of intervention for young drug misusers with complex care needs.

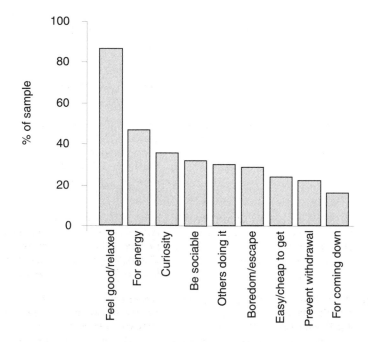

Figure 3.4 Reasons for taking drugs among young regular drug users in Ayrshire, Scotland.

From the available epidemiological data, the tiers should have the resources to deal with the populations shown in Table 3.4, although the statistics for current provision are not easy to ascertain.

Conclusion

In so far as epidemiological studies record and describe the extent of substance misuse over time, a degree of progress has been made. Despite methodological difficulties, which make comparability between regions and countries problematic, a picture of the extent of substance misuse among young people is emerging. It has proved possible to track changes in prevalence between different cohorts. However, there is still a need for standardised questions or assessment tools that allow greater comparability across national and international studies, and for

Table 3.4 Framework for integration of epidemiological methods and provision of services

Definitions	Estimates of consumption and/or criteria	Population on which estimates are likely to be based	Types of survey	Service framework
Use/misuse	Quantity/ frequency	General popu-lation; school surveys	Office of National Statistics (ONS); General Household Survey (GHS); British Crime Survey (BCS); European ESPAD	Tier 1
Use/misuse	Quantity/ frequency – 'regular' use	General popu-lation; school surveys	Office of National Statistics (ONS); General Household Survey (GHS); British Crime Survey (BCS); European ESPAD	Tier 2
Harmful use	Harmful use, dependence criteria accord-ing to ICD–10	General medical, criminal justice and social services	Home Office Addicts Index (HOAI); Regional Drug Misuse Databases (RDMDs)	Tier 3 – specialist multi-disciplinary services
Dependence	Dependence criteria accord-ing to ICD–10	Clinical treatment populations attending specialist services	Treatment popu-lations attending specialist services	Tier 4 – intensive, very special-ised services

techniques for estimating drug use among particular groups, for example those not at school. It is imperative to undertake very large longitudinal studies to complement cross-sectional studies.

Although more data than ever have accumulated, what the value in terms of reducing substance misuse has been requires careful consideration. Epidemiological studies alone cannot determine for what reasons, or 'why', and by what mechanisms, or 'how', substance misuse develops. What are the links between the wider economic and social environment, individual predisposition, and peer, family and neighbourhood influences, that affect the substance misuse statistics? By using the combination of multi-disciplinary approaches, which have both qualitative and quantitative components, epidemiological data may be better understood. Only in this way will it be possible to identify with a measure of confidence the sequence of events leading to serious substance misuse, complications of substance misuse or, indeed, the spontaneous cessation of use.

References

Abraham, M. D., Cohen, P. D. A., van Til, M. R. J., *et al* (1998) *Licit and Illicit Drug Use in the Netherlands 1997.* Amsterdam: Centrum voor Drugsonderzoek.

Aldridge, J., Parker, H. & Measham, F. (1999) *Drug Trying and Drug Use Across Adolescence: A longitudinal Study of Young People's Drug Taking in Two Regions of Northern England.* London: Drug Prevention Advisory Service, Home Office.

American Psychiatric Association (1994) *Diagnostic and Statistical Manual of Mental Disorders* (4th edn) (DSM–IV). Washington, DC: American Psychiatric Association.

Anthony, J., Warner, L. & Kessler, R. (1994) Comparative epidemiology of dependence on tobacco, alcohol, controlled substances and inhalants: basic findings from the National Comorbidity Survey. *Experimental and Clinical Psychopharmacology*, **2**, 244–268.

Awiah, J., Butt, S. & Dorn, N. (1990) The last place I would go: black people and drug services in Britain. *Druglink*, **5**, 14–15.

Bridgwood, A. (2000) *Living in Britain: Results from the 1998 General Household Survey.* London: Stationery Office.

Calafat, A., Bohrn, K., Juan, M., *et al* (1999) *Night Life in Europe and Recreative Drug Use.* Valencia: IREFREA, European Commission.

Center on Addiction and Substance Abuse (CASA) (2002) *Teen Tipplers: America's Underage Drinking Epidemic.* At http://www.casacolumbia.org newsletter1457_show.htm?doc_id=103329

Davies, J. B. (1992) *The Myth of Addiction.* Switzerland: Harwood Academic.

Department of Health (1999) *Statistics From the Regional Drug Misuse Databases for Six Months Ending March 1998.* London: Stationery Office.

—— (2000) *Statistics From the Regional Drug Misuse Databases for Six Months Ending October 2000.* London: Stationery Office.

Ditton, J. & Frischer, M. (2001) Computerised projection of future heroin epidemics: a necessity for the 21st century? *Journal of Substance Use and Abuse*, **36**, 151–166.

Frischer, M. (1996) *Estimating the Prevalence of Drug Misuse in Scotland: A Critical Review and Practical Guide.* Edinburgh: Scottish Office.

——, Hickman, H., Kraus, L., *et al* (2001) A comparison of different methods for estimating the prevalence of problematic drug misuse in Great Britain. *Addiction*, **96**, 1465–1476.

Gallacher, P. & Gray, A. G. (2002) It costs twice as much to turn Scots into an advert for healthy living. *The Scotsman*, 27 March 2002.

Ghodse, H. (2002) *Drugs and Addictive Behaviour*. Oxford: Blackwell Science.

Griffin, J. (1992) *Drug Misuse*. London: Office of Health Economics.

Harvard School of Public Health (2002) Risk factors for death and disability. In *The Global Burden of Disease and Injury Series* (executive summary). At http://www.hsph.harvard.edu/organizations/bdu/gbdsum/gbdsum5.pdf

Hawkins, J. D., Graham, J. W., Maguin, E., *et al* (2000) Exploring the effects of age of alcohol use initiation and psychosocial risk factors on subsequent alcohol misuse. *Journal of Studies on Alcohol*, **68**, 684–696.

Health Advisory Service (1996) *Children and Young People Substance Misuse Services: The Substance of Young Needs*. Norwich: HMSO.

—— (2001) *Children and Young People Substance Misuse Services: The Substance of Young Needs Review 2001*. London: Drug Prevention Advisory Service.

Hibbell, B., Andersson, B., Bjarnason, T., *et al* (1997) *The 1995 ESPAD Report*. Stockholm: Swedish Council for Information on Alcohol and Other Drugs (CAN), Council of Europe Pompidou Group.

——, ——, Ahlstrom, S., *et al* (1999) *The 1999 ESPAD Report: Alcohol and Other Drug Use Among Students in 30 European Countries*. Stockholm: Swedish Council for Information on Alcohol and Other Drugs (CAN), Council of Europe Pompidou Group.

Hofler, M., Lieb, R., Perkonigg, A., *et al* (1999) Covariates of cannabis use progression in a representative population sample of adolescents: a prospective examination of vulnerability and risk factors. *Addiction*, **94**, 1679–1694.

Interdepartmental Committee on Addiction (Brain Committee) (1965) *Second Report of the Interdepartmental Committee on Addiction (Brain Committee)*. London: HMSO.

Lawrie, P. (1978) *Drugs: Medical, Psychological and Social Facts*. London: Penguin.

Leitner, M., Shapland, J. & Wiles, P. (1993) *Drug Usage and Drug Prevention: The Views and Habits of the General Public*. London: HMSO.

Lilienfeld, D. & Stolley, P. (1994) *Foundations of Epidemiology*. Oxford: Oxford University Press.

Lloyd, C. & Joyce, R. (1999) Teaching in the tender years. *Drug and Alcohol Findings*, **1**, 4–8.

LocateNet (Web Based Drug Education Database) (2001) *Evaluated Drug Education and Prevention in Schools*. London: Drugscope.

London Health Observatory (2003) *Drug Use in London*. At http://www.lho.org.uk/hil/drug.htm#top

Kraus, L., Simon, R., Bauernfeind, R., *et al* (1998) *Study to Obtain Comparable National Estimates of Problem Drug Use: Prevalence for all EU Member States. Report on Behalf of the EMCDDA*. Lisbon: EMCDDA.

McArdle, P., Wiegersma, A., Gilvarry, E., *et al* (2000) International variations in drug use. *European Addiction Research*, **6**, 163–169.

——, ——, ——, *et al* (2002) Family structure and function and youth drug use. *Addiction*, **97**, 329–336.

National Centre for Social Research & the National Foundation for Educational Research (2001) *Smoking, Drinking and Drug Use Among Young People in England in 2000*. London: National Statistics. At http://www.official-documents.co.uk/document/doh/sddyp/survey.htm

Office of Her Majesty's Chief Inspector of Schools (2000) Drug education in schools: an update. London: Crown Office.

Parker, H., Aldridge, J. & Measham, F. (1998) *Illegal Leisure: The Normalisation of Adolescent Recreational Drug Use*. London: Routledge.

Perkonnig, A., Lieb, R., Hofler, M., *et al* (1999) Patterns of cannabis use, abuse and dependence over time: incidence, progression and stability in a sample of 1228 adolescents. *Addiction*, **94**, 1663–1678.

Plant, M. & Plant, M. (2001) Heavy drinking by young British women gives cause for concern. *British Medical Journal*, **323**, 1183.

Ramsey, M. & Partridge, S. (1999) *Drug Misuse Declared in 1998: Results From the British Crime Survey*. London: Home Office.

—— & Percy, A. (1996) Drug misuse declared: results of the 1994 British Crime Survey. London: Home Office.

——, Baker, P., Goulden, G., et al (2001) *Drug Misuse Declared in 2000: Results for the British Crime Survey*. London: Home Office.

Rutter, M. & Smith, D. (1995) *Psychosocial Disorders in Young People*. London: Academia Europaea.

Shaffer, D., Fisher, P., Dulcan, M., et al (1996) The NIMH Diagnostic Interview Schedule for Children Version 2.3 (DISC 2.3): description, acceptability, prevalence rates, and performance in the MECA study. *Journal of the American Academy of Child and Adolescent Psychiatry*, **35**, 865–877.

Sutherland, I. & Shepherd, J. P. (2001) The prevalence of alcohol, cigarette and illicit drug use in a stratified sample of English adolescents. *Addiction*, **96**, 637–640.

Taylor, A., Frischer, M., Farquhar, D. (1997) Behavioural Patterns of Illicit Substance Users in Ayrshire and Arran. Glasgow: Scottish Centre for Infection and Environmental Health.

United Kingdom Anti-drugs Coordinator (2001) *Annual Report 2000/01: A Report on Progress Since 2000 of the Government's Ten-Year Anti-drugs Strategy*. London: Home Office.

West, P., Sweeting, H. & Ecob, R. (1999) Family and friends' influences on the uptake of regular smoking from mid-adolescence to early adulthood. *Addiction*, **94**, 1397–1411.

World Health Organization (1992) *ICD–10 Classification of Mental and Behavioural Disorders*.World Health Organization: Geneva.

Zoccolillo, M., Vitaro, F. & Tremblay, R. E. (1999) Problem drug and alcohol use in a community sample of adolescents. *Journal of the American Academy of Child and Adolescent Psychiatry*, **38**, 900–907.

CHAPTER 4

Determinants of substance misuse

Paul McArdle and John Macleod

Key points

- For most young people, peer use approaches the status of a necessary condition for drug use and misuse. This may be due to the access to drugs facilitated by some peer groups.
- Attention-deficit hyperactivity disorder is a common antecedent of substance misuse in young people, especially if it persists through adolescence. In part this may be because of its impulsive, risk-taking component.
- Family adversity may act by loosening the ties to adults and increasing ties to peer groups and by predisposing to conduct disorder.
- Problematic family relationships may be more influential than family structure.
- Conduct disordered children and young people are at particularly high risk of substance misuse. This is often because their relationships with adults in the family and at school are poor, and because they affiliate with like-minded peers.

Introduction

This chapter explores the origins of youth substance misuse, in particular the influence of development, both normal and abnormal, on substance use and misuse. It also aims to describe how the interplay of developmental characteristics, social environment and culture may lead to substance misuse.

Normal and abnormal development

A developmental perspective means a 'dynamic view ... knowing what led ... to [in this case substance misuse], the network of changes in which it is nested, and its later manifestations' (Sroufe, 1995). The so-called developmental tasks of adolescence include the capacity to cope actively with a series of more or less universal changes. The most obvious of these are the physical changes of puberty, the different gender relationships, and the greater autonomy from the family, as well as the greater requirement to plan, to forge relationships outside the family and to distinguish those who are likely to be supportive from others. The ability to plan, the increasing capacity to organise life around realistic goals, may be a crucial marker of mature functioning in adolescence (Quinton & Rutter, 1985). Related abilities include those to work, to reflect and to cope with adversity. These characteristics emerge from childhood precursors: the experience of secure attachment, of success in social, scholastic or other areas (and hence self-efficacy), of safe exploration of childhood friendships and of play. They also reflect normal integrated cognitive and affective development. Ultimately, they lead to young adults capable of productive work, raising children and sustaining relationships.

The relevant literature draws on the fields of child development and psychopathology. This requires some familiarity with disorders such as attention-deficit hyperactivity disorder and conduct disorder, and with concepts such as attachment that are relatively new to the adult literature. Conduct disorder is characterised by 'a repetitive and persistent pattern of dissocial, aggressive, or defiant conduct' (World Health Organization, 1992). It tends to emerge from situations of 'ineffective ... coercive or hostile parenting, abuse and neglect ... and poor supervision'. It is possible that the effects are mediated through social learning, 'by rewarding inappropriate behaviour and encouraging coercive behaviour patterns' (Rutter *et al*, 1998). In addition, poor quality of parenting interferes with the process of attachment by the child, in the first place to parents (Rutter *et al*, 1998). In this way, poor parenting may impair the child's capacity to develop trusting, secure relationships, initially within the family. Such impairment renders a child unable to satisfy his or her need for emotional warmth and intimacy. Consequently, deprived of the intimate bond with parents, the child is unable to avail him- or herself of the values and social conventions for which the family is a repository, or of the stimulation that is a part of family life. Furthermore, the child is troubled and angry and, because of impoverished play and sociability, cannot enjoy him- or herself in solo or sociable play. As children in this state develop, they tend to generate similar relationships with others, such as teachers. They then enter adolescence without the restraint of family or other adults, without adult values and, suspicious of the deferred variety, demand immediate satisfaction. These children are often diagnosed by child and adolescent mental health practitioners as conduct disordered.

Hence, the presence of conduct disorder may mark an early fracture in the relationship between the child and adults. Conduct disordered young people display problematic relationships, risky sexual behaviour, teenage pregnancy, school failure and drop-out, and persistent criminality (Farrington *et al*, 1990; Ary *et al*, 1999) and are at high risk for substance misuse (Gittelman *et al*, 1985; Fergusson & Woodward, 2000).

The adversities that lead to conduct disorder may be present throughout the child's development. However, change in family circumstance, such as loss of a parent through death or separation, abuse, or other family catastrophe, may precipitate a later onset but similar developmental course.

Attention-deficit hyperactivity disorder is an early-onset (often pre-school) condition, characterised by a 'persistent pattern of inattention and or hyperactivity/impulsivity that is more frequent and severe than is typically observed in individuals at a comparable level of development' (American Psychiatric Association, 1994). These children are at greater risk than others of accidents and school failure. Many of these children also display other developmental vulnerabilities, such as minor physical anomalies (Arsenault *et al*, 2000), clumsiness, specific learning disabilities (Rasmussen & Gillberg, 2000) and developmental language disorders (Beitchman *et al*, 2001). Genetic factors may also be of importance in the origin of these vulnerabilities (Goodman & Stevenson, 1990). Other factors such as exposure to alcohol *in utero* (Sampson *et al*, 1997; Yates *et al*, 1998), low birth weight and other forms of perinatal adversity (Stenninger *et al*, 1998) or severe early deprivation (O'Connor & Rutter, 2000) may contribute.

Children with attention-deficit hyperactivity disorder are not easy to raise, not least because of their accident proneness (Bijur *et al*, 1986) and consequent increased need for supervision, as well as the complaints of schools and neighbours. Despite the ameliorating effects of maturation, some of their parents will display similar characteristics to the children, and may be vulnerable themselves. A child-rearing environment that is often fraught, critical or emotionally unsupportive arises. Therefore, even when their families are striving to care for them and to raise them responsibly, these children are also at enhanced risk of conduct disorder (McArdle *et al*, 1995).

Links between child development and substance use and misuse

Studies of youth substance use and misuse indicate a wide array of developmental and contextual correlates. However, in order to attribute a causal relationship between correlated or associated factors and substance use and misuse, certain types of evidence and several issues of interpretation must be considered. These have been discussed extensively (e.g. Hill, 1965; Rothman, 1976; Susser, 1991; Parascandola & Weed, 2001). For example, a causal influence should precede the onset of the substance use or misuse. There should also be evidence of a dose–response relationship between the putative cause and the disorder (e.g. the more cigarettes smoked, the greater the likelihood of lung disease). Confounding factors, that is influences that vary with both the cause and the consequence, must be taken into account through appropriate statistical adjustment and the limitations of such adjustment should be recognised (Phillips & Davey Smith, 1991). An illustration of confounding can be found in the association between perinatal events and subsequent child behaviour disorder described by Pasamanick *et al* (1956). These authors attributed the latter to minimal brain damage consequent to perinatal injury or hypoxic brain damage. However, there was failure to take into account that social disadvantage correlated with both behaviour disorder and perinatal adversity, and could be an alternative explanation for the association. In addition, there should be a plausible mechanism to explain the association, although, clearly, this is dependent on the general level of under-standing of the processes under examination and plausibility alone is a poor test of a causal hypothesis (Macleod *et al*, 2001). In examining the literature, these strictures will be kept in mind.

Longitudinal studies are important in attempting to determine a sequence of events across the life span, and in helping to disentangle the direction of causality between substance misuse and other factors. For instance, Boyle *et al* (1993) used longitudinal data from a large repre-sentative sample of Ontario children to examine these relationships. They showed that, of 8–12-year-olds with conduct disorder, approxi-mately 21.4% reported subsequent use of 'hard drugs' (e.g. stimulants, hallucinogens, opiates) four years later. Among those originally without conduct disorder, the corresponding rate was 3.7%. In addition, there was a linear relationship between the number of conduct disorder symptoms (aggression, running away, defiance, truancy, vandalism and theft) identified by teachers and subsequent hard drug use. The same group also demonstrated that conduct disorder in early adolescence predicted later poly-drug use, after they controlled statistically for prior substance use in early adolescence (Boyle *et al*, 1992).

The Christchurch Child Health and Development Study followed 1265 children from birth to young adulthood. It, too, showed a linear relationship between different degrees of 'attentional difficulties' (key symptoms of attention-deficit hyperactivity disorder) in childhood and the likelihood of 'alcohol misuse/dependence' and 'other substance misuse/dependence' at 18 years (Fergusson & Lynskey, 1997). The former ranged from 17% to 33% and the latter from 8% to 26% (a similar figure to that reported in Ontario for use of 'hard drugs' among previously conduct disordered children), depending on the rated severity of initial 'attentional difficulties'. In a study of 717 low-birth weight children, Chilcoat & Breslau (1999) reported that, among those without childhood behaviour problems (attention-deficit hyperactivity disorder or symptoms of conduct disorder) at the age of six years, the rate of adolescent use of psychoactive substances was 17%. Among those with attention-deficit hyperactivity disorder it rose to 29%, and among those with combined attention-deficit hyperactivity disorder and moderate conduct problems it rose to 40%.

These studies focus on use or indirect measures of misuse because the numbers displaying more problematic forms of misuse are relatively small and data gathering is often reliant on questionnaires that do not fully assess 'harm' associated with misuse. An examination of harm and dependent use requires a fuller assessment of respondents and often the tracking of high-risk groups. For instance, Gittelman *et al* (1985) compared the long-term outcome of a clinical sample, originally referred because of childhood hyperactivity, and controls, who were referred by paediatricians and not hyperactive. They showed that 19% of the hyperactive children followed up at a mean age of 18.3 years had a substance use disorder, compared with 7% of the controls. Among those with persisting hyperactivity at follow-up, the rate of substance use disorder was 32%. Among those who additionally developed conduct disorder, the rate was 59%. The onset of conduct disorder *never* followed the onset of substance use disorder. It occurred contemporaneously in approximately 20% and preceded the onset of substance use disorder in the other 80% of cases. The pattern of findings was similar irrespective of whether the substance misused was illicit drugs or alcohol.

In another form of a high-risk study, but using a retrospective methodology, Robins & McEvoy (1990) reported on links between adult substance misuse and subject-recalled child conduct disorder. Using the Epidemiologic Catchment Area (ECA) data-set of 20 000 adults, they found that, among respondents who had ever used illicit drugs, 26% reported childhood conduct disorder, compared with 11% among those who had never used illicit drugs. Among those who had used illicit drugs, any symptom of conduct disorder in childhood (e.g. theft, truancy, fighting, vandalism) was associated with at least a doubled risk of substance use disorder, compared with those reporting no symptoms of conduct disorder. They were also able to estimate the 'population attributable risk' (PAR) attached to each symptom, which was 49% in respect of stealing. This means that, among those who had used an illicit substance, stealing identified 'half of those who would develop serious substance misuse (those with consequent problems in at least three areas of their lives)'. This was much greater than the PAR of 11% linked with conduct disorder alone (Boyle *et al*, 1993). Furthermore, Robins & McEvoy (1990) reported a linear relationship between the number of conduct problems reported in childhood and the rate of subsequent adult substance misuse. The rates for 'ever' used drugs ranged from 2% among those without childhood symptoms of conduct disorder to 56% among those with eight childhood symptoms of conduct disorder. This figure is very similar to that reported by Gittelman *et al* (1985).

Other longitudinal studies have examined somewhat different constructs of childhood adjustment. For instance, Newcomb & Bentler (1990) reported on findings from an eight-year follow-up of 654 young adolescents in a representative community sample. They created variables of 'social conformity' – approximately the converse of conduct disorder – 'academic orientation', 'emotional distress' and 'drug use' on the basis of self-reports at three time points. Using a path analysis model, social conformity at time 1 (early adolescence) was significantly, and negatively, associated with drug use at time 1 and at time 2 (when it was statistically independent of the effect of drug use at time 1). However, drug use at either time did not predict, positively or negatively, social conformity at time 2: degrees of social conformity predicted drug use, not vice versa.

Masse & Tremblay (1997) reported an evaluation of the prognostic importance of three personality dimensions: harm avoidance, high novelty seeking, and reward dependence. These 'neuro-genetic' traits were hypothesised by Cloninger (1987) to underlie so-called type 2 alcoholism. They obtained teacher data when the subjects were aged six years and self-report substance use data when they were 11, 12, 13, 14 and 15 years old. Personality constructs were 'inferred' from teacher questionnaires. 'Novelty seeking' was identified using a questionnaire item that checked for 'restless, runs about or jumps up and down and does not keep still, squirmy and fidgety'. These closely resemble DSM–IV symptoms of attention-deficit hyperactivity disorder (American Psychiatric Association, 1994). Harm avoidance was indicated by 'worries ... afraid of new situations', which could be perceived as the opposite of the DSM–IV impulsivity component of attention-deficit hyperactivity disorder. They reported that high novelty seeking and low harm avoidance at age six years significantly predicted alcohol, drug and cigarette use in adolescence at all follow-up data points.

Taken as a whole, symptoms of childhood behaviour disorder, whether attention-deficit hyperactivity disorder or conduct disorder, precede substance misuse. However, substance misuse does not precede conduct disorder. Also, there is a 'dose–response' relationship between the number of symptoms and the likelihood of subsequent substance misuse. These findings are consistent with the existence of a causal link.

Family structure and relationships

There are also relevant findings from cross-sectional studies, especially those that attempt to control for confounding factors. For instance, Miller (1997) demonstrated an association between family disadvantage, identified by single-parent status, and youth drug use. However, the significance of this association disappeared when individual 'delinquent' behaviour was taken into account. In another recent European study, McArdle *et al* (2000) demonstrated that family influences, marked by single-parent status or reconstituted family, predicted drug use independently of self-reported delinquent behaviour. However, the latter was by far the most important predictor of drug use. Of family variables, the quality of the parent–child relationship rather than family structure appears to be the most important influence (McArdle *et al*, 2002*a*).

Genetic factors

Kendler *et al* (2000) demonstrated that the monozygotic exceeded the dizygotic concordance for drug use, heavy use, misuse and dependence in a large sample of US twins. Genetic effects were greater for heavy use, misuse or dependence than for 'use'. These data raise the question of what constitutes the phenotype – or endophenotype, which 'reflects processes more proximal to gene expression than the clinical phenotype' (Kendler, 2001). For example, in the absence of drug availability, what would this look like? In keeping with the cross-sectional and longitudinal data, Cadoret *et al* (1995) demonstrated 'a circuitous route through antisocial personality disorder in the biologic parent ... intervening variables of adoptee aggressivity, conduct disorder, antisocial personality disorder ... [to] drug misuse/dependency'. Genetic studies have also demonstrated substantial shared environmental effects relevant to the development of substance misuse (Han *et al*, 1999). This may be linked to parental substance misuse, family adversity and exposure to substances in the community.

Peer group factors

The role of peers in promoting drug use has proved an important area of research. However, Bauman & Ennett (1996) have argued that earlier research tended to exaggerate the influence of peers. This view originates from the tendency of vulnerable young people to select like-minded peers, so that affiliation and drug use may derive from a third factor, for instance a shared predisposition to drug use. Others have argued that the influence of peers is statistically independent (Herting *et al*, 1996; Hofler *et al*, 1999). However, in the longitudinal Christchurch

Child Health and Development Study, conduct problems at 13 years predicted both deviant peer affiliations at 18 years and drug misuse/dependence. The authors concluded that deviant peer affiliations represent 'an intervening variable' on a pathway between symptoms of conduct disorder and substance misuse/dependence (Fergusson & Woodward, 2000). Hence, the association between deviant peer affiliations and drug misuse derives, at least in part, from the association between them both and a third variable, antecedent conduct problems or disorder. Nevertheless, irrespective of personal predisposition, it is likely that the availability of drugs through peer groups is virtually a necessary condition for drug use and misuse.

Adverse life events

The roles of other potentially formative experiences in the development of substance misuse have been assessed. These include, for instance, physical and sexual abuse (Bulik et al, 2001) and family violence (Fergusson & Horwood, 1998). However, individual stressors such as maltreatment or inter-parental violence tend to occur in the context of pervasive disadvantage and family disruption. When this is taken into account, the predictive value of individual stressors declines or disappears. It is likely that this occurs because the elements of family dysfunction strongly correlate together and, crucially, with poor quality of parenting (Rutter et al, 1998).

Conclusion

This chapter focuses on the origin of substance misuse rather than occasional or experimental use. It is likely that peer influences and particularly availability, rather than personal vulnerability, loom larger in the causality of occasional use. However, the findings suggest causal chains linking personal vulnerability (e.g. attention-deficit hyperactivity disorder and conduct disorder) to substance misuse. Conduct disorder in particular marks weakened ties to adult support and values. Substance availability facilitated by the peer group completes the chain of causality leading to substance misuse. Such a developmental chain, invoking a dynamic interplay between biological and environmental factors, is analogous to our emerging understanding in other areas of dysfunction and ill health. For instance, low birth weight may combine with low educational attainment in enhancing risk for coronary heart disease (e.g. Barker et al, 2001). However, even among those with apparently high degrees of predisposition and adverse environments, some individuals do not develop substance misuse. Furthermore, since some are likely to develop substance misuse without conduct disorder, the population with attributable risk will be well short of 100%. Improved understanding is required of the mechanisms whereby protective factors operate (those that are not simply the absence of risk factors), as well as of the non-conduct-disordered pathways to drug misuse.

References

American Psychiatric Association (1994) *Diagnostic and Statistical Manual of Mental Disorders* (4th edn) (DSM–IV). Washington, DC: American Psychiatric Association.

Arseneault, L., Tremblay, R. E., Boulerice, B., *et al* (2000) Minor physical anomalies and family adversity as risk factors for violent delinquency in adolescence. *American Journal of Psychiatry*, **157**, 917–923.

Ary, D., Duncan, T., Biglan, A., *et al* (1999) Development of adolescent problem behaviour. *Journal of Abnormal Child Psychology*, **27**, 141–150.

Barker, D., Forsen, T., Uutela, A., *et al* (2001) Size at birth and resilience to effects of poor living conditions in adult life: longitudinal study. *British Medical Journal*, **323**, 1273–1276.

Bauman, K. & Ennett, S. (1996) On the importance of peer influence for adolescent drug use: commonly neglected considerations. *Addiction*, **91**, 185–198.

Beitchman, J. H., Wilson, B., Johnson, C. J., *et al* (2001) Fourteen-year follow-up of speech/language-impaired and control children: psychiatric outcome. *Journal of the American Academy of Child and Adolescent Psychiatry*, **40**, 75–82.

Bijur, P. E., Stewart-Brown, S. & Butler, N. (1986) Child behaviour and accidental injury in 11,966 preschoolchildren. *American Journal of Diseases of Childhood*, **140**, 487–492.

Boyle, M., Offord, D., Racine, Y., *et al* (1992) Predicting substance use in late adolescence: results from the Ontario Child Health Study Follow-up. *American Journal of Psychiatry*, **149**, 761–767.

— , — , — , *et al* (1993) Predicting substance use in early adolescence based on parent and teacher assessments of childhood psychiatric disorder: results from the Ontario Child Health Study Follow-up. *Journal of Child Psychology and Psychiatry*, **34**, 535–544.

Bulik, C., Prescott, C. & Kendler, K. (2001) Features of child sexual misuse and the development of psychiatric and substance use disorders. *British Journal of Psychiatry*, **179**, 444–450.

Cadoret, R., Yates, W., Troughton, E., *et al* (1995) Genetic–environmental interaction in the genesis of aggressivity and conduct disorders. *Archives of General Psychiatry*, **52**, 916–924.

Chilcoat, H. D. & Breslau, N. (1999) Pathways from ADHD to early drug use. *Journal of the American Academy of Child and Adolescent Psychiatry*, **38**, 1347–1354.

Cloninger, C. (1987) Neurogenetic adaptive mechanisms in alcoholism. *Science*, **236**, 410–416.

Farrington, A., Loeber, R. & Van Kammen, W. (1990) Long-term criminal outcomes of hyperactivity-impulsivity-attention-deficit and conduct problems in childhood. In *Straight and Devious Pathways from Childhood to Adulthood* (eds L. Robins & M. Rutter), pp. 62–81. Cambridge: Cambridge University Press.

Fergusson, D. & Horwood, L. (1998) Exposure to interparental violence in childhood and psychosocial adjustment in young adulthood. *Child Misuse and Neglect*, **22**, 339–357.

— & Lynskey, M. (1997) Physical punishment/maltreatment during childhood and adjustment in young adulthood. *Child Misuse and Neglect*, **21**, 617–630.

— & Woodward, L. (2000) Educational, psychosocial and early sexual outcomes of girls with conduct problems in early adolescence. *Journal of Child Psychology and Psychiatry*, **41**, 779–792.

Gittelman, R., Mannuzza, S., Shenker, R., *et al* (1985) Hyperactive boys almost grown up 1: psychiatric status. *Archives of General Psychiatry*, **42**, 937–947.

Goodman, R. & Stevenson, J. (1990) A twin study of hyperactivity: 1. An examination of hyperactivity scores and categories derived from Rutter teacher and parent questionnaires. *Journal of Child Psychology and Psychiatry*, **30**, 671–689.

Han, C., McGue, M. & Iacono, W. (1999) Lifetime tobacco, alcohol and other substance use in adolescent Minnesota twins: univariate and multivariate behavioral genetic analyses. *Addiction*, **94**, 981–993.

Herting, J., Eggert, L. & Thompson, E. (1996) A multidimensional model of adolescent drug involvement. *Journal of Research on Adolescence*, **6**, 325–361.

Hill, A. B. (1965) The environment and disease: association or causation? *Proceedings of the Royal Society of Medicine*, **58**, 295–300.

Hofler, M., Leib, R., Perkonigg, A., *et al* (1999) Covariates of cannabis use progression in a representative sample of adolescents: a prospective examination of vulnerability and risk factors. *Addiction*, **94**, 1679–1694.

Kendler, K. (2001) Twin studies of psychiatric illness: an update. *Archives of General Psychiatry*, **58**, 1005–1014.

Kendler, K., Karkowski, L., Neale, M., *et al* (2000) Illicit psychoactive substance use, heavy use, abuse and dependence in a US population-based sample of male twins. *Archives of General Psychiatry*, **57**, 261–269.

Macleod, J., Davey Smith, G., Heslop, P., *et al* (2001) Are the effects of psychosocial exposures attributable to confounding? Evidence from a prospective observational study on psychological stress and mortality. *Journal of Epidemiology and Community Health*, **55**, 878–884.

Masse, L. & Tremblay, R. (1997) Behavior of boys in kindergarten and the onset of substance use during adolescence. *Archives of General Psychiatry*, **54**, 62–68.

McArdle, P., O'Brien, G. & Kolvin, I. (1995) Hyperactivity: prevalence and relationship with conduct disorder. *Journal of Child Psychology and Psychiatry*, **36**, 279–305.

— , Wiegersma, A., Gilvarry, E., *et al* (2000) International variations in drug use: the effect of individual behaviours, peer and family influences and geographical location. *European Addiction Research*, **6**, 163–169.

— , — , — , *et al* (2002*a*) European adolescent substance use: the roles of family structure, function and gender. *Addiction*, **97**, 329–336.

— , Moseley, D., Quibell, T., *et al* (2002*b*) School-based indicated prevention: a randomised trial of group therapy. *Journal of Clinical Psychology and Psychiatry*, **43**, 705–715.

Miller, P. (1997) Family structure, personality, drinking, smoking and illicit drug use: a study of UK teenagers. *Drug and Alcohol Dependence*, **45**, 121–129.

Newcomb, M. & Bentler, P. (1990) Antecedents and consequences of cocaine use: an eight year study from early adolescence to young adulthood. In *Straight and Devious Pathways from Childhood to Adulthood* (eds L. Robins & M. Rutter), pp. 158–181. Cambridge: Cambridge University Press.

O'Connor, T. & Rutter, M. (2000) Attachment disorder behavior following early severe deprivation: extension and longitudinal follow-up: English and Romanian Adoptees Study Team. *Journal of the American Academy of Child and Adolescent Psychiatry*, **39**, 703–712.

Parascandola, M. & Weed, D. L. (2001) Causation in epidemiology. *Journal of Epidemiology and Community Health*, **55**, 905–912.

Pasamanick, B., Knobloch, H. & Lilienfield, A. (1956) Socioeconomic status and some precursors of neuropsychiatric disorder. *American Journal of Orthopsychiatry*, **26**, 594–601.

Phillips, A. N. & Davey Smith, G. (1991) How independent are 'independent' effects? Relative risk estimation when correlated exposures are measured imprecisely. *Journal of Clinical Epidemiology*; **44**, 1223–1231.

Quinton, D. & Rutter, M. (1985) Parenting behaviour of mothers raised in care. In *Longitudinal Studies in Child Psychology and Psychiatry* (ed. A. R. Nicol), pp. 157–203. Chichester: Wiley.

Rasmussen, P. & Gillberg, C. (2000) Natural outcome of ADHD with developmental coordination disorder at age 22 years: a controlled longitudinal community based study. *Journal of the American Academy of Child and Adolescent Psychiatry*, **39**, 1424–1431.

Robins, L. & McEvoy, L. (1990) Conduct problems as predictors of substance misuse. In *Straight and Devious Pathways from Childhood to Adulthood* (eds L. Robins & M. Rutter), pp. 182–204. Cambridge: Cambridge University Press.

Rothman, K. J. (1976) Causes. *American Journal of Epidemiology*; **104**, 587–592.

Rutter, M., Giller, H. & Hagell, A. (1998) *Antisocial Behavior by Young People*. Cambridge: Cambridge University Press.

Sampson, P. D., Streissguth, A. P., Bookstein, F. L., *et al* (1997) Incidence of fetal alcohol syndrome and prevalence of alcohol-related neurodevelopmental disorder. *Teratology*, **56**, 317–326.

Sroufe, L. A. (1995) *Emotional Development: The Organisation of Emotional Life in the Early Years*. Cambridge: Cambridge University Press.

Stenninger, E., Flink, R., Eriksson, B., *et al* (1998) Long-term neurological dysfunction and neonatal hypoglycaemia after diabetic pregnancy. *Archives of Disease in Childhood: Fetal and Neonatal Edition*, **79**, F174–179.

Susser, M. (1991) What is a cause and how do we know one? A grammar for pragmatic epidemiology. *American Journal of Epidemiology*, **133**, 635–648.

World Health Organization (1992) *ICD–10 Classification of Mental and Behavioural Disorders*. Geneva: World Health Organisation.

Yates, W. R., Cadoret, R. J., Troughton, E. P., *et al* (1998) Effect of fetal alcohol exposure on adult symptoms of nicotine, alcohol, and drug dependence. *Alcoholism: Clinical and Experimental Research*, **22**, 914–920.

CHAPTER 5

Social influences

Daphne Rumball and Ilana B. Crome

Key points

- Social antecedents and consequences are not readily defined as causes and effects owing to the complex interactions of substance use and the environment. Studies indicate a high level of social disadvantage among young substance users. Social factors have a major influence on the course of substance use through psychological and other mechanisms.
- Some social influences are protective. These factors can be strengthened as strategies for prevention and as components of treatment.
- Social complications of substance use have a major impact on physical and emotional health in addition to the direct effects of the substance use itself.
- Sexual exploitation has strong correlations with substance use – both as a risk factor and as a consequence. Difficulties related to sexual orientation also predispose to substance use. These aspects of young people's social experience should be a focus of careful assessment and intervention.
- Attention to all aspects of social influence, including education and training, housing, relationships and criminality, is essential for effective treatment interventions and requires a skilled, multi-disciplinary and multi-agency approach.

Introduction: substance use as an aspect of risk taking

Adolescence is a time for experimentation and risk taking. Adolescent development includes behaviours that are counter to adult advice and social conventions. At the same time, adolescent behaviour is greatly influenced by a desire to conform to peer norms, to be 'cool' and in touch with the latest thinking and activities. Therefore, any attempt by professionals and parents to influence behaviour in the direction of risk reduction, harm minimisation and the avoidance of complications may face a considerable challenge. In this context, it is almost self-evident that some adolescent risk taking or group conformity will lead to substance use, and will, concomitantly, have social complications. It is important to recognise these common factors and to avoid attributing all social morbidity to a direct effect of substance use. As discussed in Chapters 4 and 6, the observed comorbidity is likely to arise from common predisposing factors.

Since there are very few robust prospective studies on these issues, we have found it almost impossible clearly to separate cause and effect, and prefer, therefore, to describe associations, relationships and influences. Clinical experience, however, does provide a degree of information about temporal associations and directions in the development of substance problems, but one must be extremely cautious about ascribing causality.

Nevertheless, once substance misuse has been established, clinical experience and research suggest that further social harms accrue (Ellickson et al, 2001; Guo et al, 2001). Studies of young substance users indicate a high rate of social disadvantage, much of which resolves with the holistic treatment of the substance problem (Crome et al, 2000). It is not surprising that the best outcomes require a combined social, psychological and medical approach (Marsden et al, 2000). The notion that removal of the substance that appears to have generated social harms will lead to the removal of those harms is not supported by experience; the social problems themselves tend to heighten the risk of substance use and to make its resolution more problematic.

The antecedents of substance use, and the later social, physical and psychological complications, may lead to complex social problems very quickly. Young substance users are vulnerable to exploitation, particularly if they are homeless, have a learning disability or are mentally ill. The presence of coercive adults, sexual exploitation, parental neglect or severe behavioural problems indicates the need for a multi-agency child protection framework when caring for adolescents (Health Advisory Service, 2001) and occasionally the need for formal child protection. Young substance misusers may themselves be parents, as many of the risk factors for substance misuse are common with those for teenage pregnancy.

The use of substances before it is legal to do so, illicit substance use, the use of substances while inexperienced, and heavy use of legal substances are all subject to risk. The complications are physical, emotional, legal and social. Complications in any one of these domains may lead indirectly to further social predicaments. For example, poor mental health may contribute to difficulty gaining or retaining employment or housing, and physical illness may lead to social disadvantage and be exacerbated by the resultant poverty.

For some young people, risk taking itself is attractive. Others – those with low social expectations and those who find the pleasure of substance use outweighs the potential problems – may be indifferent to the possibility of complications (Nowinski, 1990). Interventions that emphasise negative outcomes of substance use may therefore be unhelpful.

Premorbid social risk factors

Environmental and cultural factors

Environmental factors associated with adolescent substance use include neighbourhood crime, poverty and a lack of community support structures (Brook & Brook, 1990). Within the context of these factors there are also those of culture and ethnicity. Ethnic minorities in Britain experience a high degree of social exclusion in terms of poverty, housing deprivation and educational disadvantage. All these factors are associated with problematic drug use. Members of Black and other minority groups have been significantly underrepresented among populations of drug users seeking treatment.

For example, in the London Health Observatory study, a substantially higher proportion of crack users arrested were from Black minority ethnic groups compared with crack users in treatment. Overall, among reports of people presenting to specialist drug agencies, approximately three-quarters were White and less than 10% were from Black ethnic minorities. In contrast, among reports of people assessed in police stations, less than 60% were White and 24% were from Black minority ethnic groups (London Health Observatory, 2003). These figures suggest that minority groups are at greater risk of arrest but obtain lower rates of access to treatment despite the national policy of arrest referral for drug users. Language and cultural needs are often neglected and there is little outreach to help to address social and cultural barriers to service access.

Family relationships

Adverse family factors can set the scene for criminality, social problems and psychiatric complications, as well as being formative in the development of substance use itself (Stoker & Swadi, 1990). Early age of onset of alcohol and nicotine use, the major predictors of further substance use (Best et al, 2000), are greatly influenced by family behaviour. One-third of divorces, 40% of domestic violence and 20% of child abuse cases are associated with substance misuse.

Family conflict, poor and inconsistent parenting, the use of substances by parents, and attitudes favourable to substance use are all associated with an increased prevalence of adolescent use. Domestic violence has an adverse effect on children's experience of family life and on the development of self-esteem. As a result, there is an increased prevalence of post-traumatic stress disorder and conduct disorder (Emery *et al*, 1982), both of which are associated with an increased risk of adolescent substance use and self-harm.

Peer relationships

Rutter (1985) found that resilient children have a repertoire of problem-solving skills and a belief in their own self-efficacy. Association with peers who use drugs is unsurprisingly linked with an increased risk of personal use. However, this may be mitigated by external support systems which encourage positive values; for example, a caring relationship with at least one adult, sport and hobbies, strong religious beliefs and a supportive peer and family environment all appear to have a protective value. Primary and secondary preventive strategies need to evaluate these observations and, if appropriate, to incorporate relevant social interventions.

Unstable housing and homelessness

Substance-using populations and homeless populations have a high prevalence of young people formerly in care. One study found that 22% of homeless people had been through the care system as young people and that two-thirds were dependent on drugs or had a hazardous drinking pattern, or both. In the age group 16–24 years, 40% had attempted suicide at some time in their lives and there was a high prevalence of mental illness (Office for National Statistics, 2000). Homelessness and substance use are also linked to high rates of unemployment.

Education, training and employment opportunities

Young people who use substances frequently attend school irregularly and may stop attending well before the official leaving age. Indeed, drug use may be the major, often unbending, reason for suspension or exclusion. Poor concentration, reading difficulties and academic failure are linked to substance use. Clinical impression suggests a high prevalence of mild learning disability, but this is an under-researched area. Precisely how these multiple factors interact, among others, with limited parental expectations as well as inadequate supervision and monitoring of schoolwork is unclear. However, the inability to obtain qualifications restricts entry into training, the workplace higher education. Low self-esteem may follow and lead to initiation into, or an increase in, substance use. On the other hand, above average intelligence and academic performance in conjunction with ongoing educational opportunities and other interests are protective (Rutter, 1985).

Emotional health

As stated earlier, substance use has many predisposing psychological factors. These may be exacerbated by the adverse consequences of alcohol and drug use. Separations, bereavements, imprisonment and assaults are associated with substance use. The development of post-traumatic stress disorder as well as the risk of self-harm and suicide are greatly increased in substance users. Psychiatric symptoms and deviance in early adolescence predict heavy alcohol use three years later (Kumpulainen, 2000). Williams & Morgan (1994) suggested that the most significant effect on adolescent suicide would be achieved by the prevention and treatment of substance use.

Adolescence is a time of sexual development, during which some young people struggle with issues of sexual orientation and identity. For young gay and lesbian people these stresses are known to be associated with an increased risk of substance use, particularly alcohol (McKirnan & Peterson, 1988; Adger, 1991). Distress and anxiety related to sexuality may not be revealed unless sympathetically explored, can remain a hidden source of ongoing problematic substance use, and are associated with an increased risk of self-harm (Ryan & Futterman, 1998).

Ethnic minorities have particular problems accessing treatment. Analysis suggests that Asian and Black patients are less likely than White patients to have their psychological problems identified in primary care settings (Odell et al, 1997). The prevalence of comorbid psychiatric illness and substance use is underrepresented in clinical settings.

Commander et al (1999) found that alcohol misuse was not recognised during routine consultations, even when the nature of the problem had known associations with alcohol. In their study of a population of 16–64-year-olds, only half of those who consulted the general practitioner had their problem identified. Case recognition was particularly poor for women, young persons and Asians. The main filter to people accessing specialist services came at the primary care level, where referral was found to be least likely for young people and ethnic minorities.

Physical health: mortality and morbidity

As discussed further in Chapter 8, poor physical health is known to have strong correlations with poverty and social deprivation, partly through accidents, dietary neglect and the failure to access primary care for prevention or treatment. There is considerable mortality associated with substance misuse. There are 120 000-smoking related deaths per year in England and Wales. Smoking accounts for 20% of deaths at all ages, and 25% of deaths between 25 and 35.

In the UK there are about 40 000 alcohol-related deaths per annum. One-quarter of road traffic fatalities have blood alcohol levels above 80 mg%, as do 30% of pedestrians sustaining injuries. Illicit drugs are found in the blood of 15–20% of drivers involved in fatal road crashes.

Alcohol affects every organ in the body and its use above recommended safe levels is associated with heart disease, liver cirrhosis, many types of cancer, and neurological as well as gastrointestinal problems. Prostitution and sexual exploitation are linked through multiple factors with substance misuse and are associated with increased risks of violence and exposure to sexually transmitted infections, thus compounding health and social risks. Crack cocaine use is common among sex workers and is linked with an increased risk of hepatitis B and C infection, and with termination of pregnancy (Ward *et al*, 2000). Alcohol is strongly related to high-risk sexual behaviour, unwanted pregnancy and sexually transmitted infections, as well as domestic violence, accidents and social disharmony. One-third of domestic accidents are associated with alcohol misuse.

Between 1000 and 3000 drug misusers died as a result of overdose in 1998 in England and Wales. The statistical uncertainty relates to problems with current databases. Compared with the general population, mortality rates are higher among addicts (standardised mortality ratio = 7). Injecting drug users have a mortality rate 12–22 times greater than their peers. As is further discussed in Chapter 6, compared with the general population, suicide rates are higher among addicts (standardised mortality ratio for males = 4.4; for females = 11.3). Overdose by accident is not always distinct from suicidal behaviour (Neale, 2000).

Involvement in criminality, especially if this results in youth custody or prison, compounds the risks to physical health through unsafe injecting behaviour and high-risk sexual activity in custody, and accidental overdose in the period immediately after release from custody.

Pregnancy, sexual exploitation and prostitution

Mental illness leading to suicide is the major cause of maternal death, and substance misuse in pregnancy is the main predisposing factor for 15% of all recorded maternal deaths by suicide in pregnancy and the perinatal period (Lewis & Drife, 2002). Young mothers who are socially disadvantaged are particularly at risk.

Pregnancy

Substance use has been shown to increase by a factor of four the rates of sexual risk taking and early, unplanned or undesired pregnancy, and to increase the risk of abortion by a factor of five (Mensch & Kandel, 1992). Substance use is often accompanied by amenorrhoea, as a result of which the young person may not realise that there is a risk of pregnancy and may not be aware of the pregnancy until quite an advanced stage. This can lead to further complications of poor antenatal care, amplifying the problems of young people, especially homeless educationally deprived substance users, in accessing health care.

Pregnant teenage women who use substances are more likely to have serious patterns of substance use and are at increased risk of physical and emotional violence (Martin *et al*, 1999). Pregnancy is associated with an increased risk of domestic violence, which commonly occurs for the first time during pregnancy (Mezey & Bewley, 1997).

Sexual exploitation and prostitution

The involvement of younger people in the sex industry should be regarded as a form of childhood sexual abuse rather than prostitution. Many criminal justice agencies in the UK now adopt this approach to all people under 18 years.

Young people at school are often overlooked in studies concerning sex for pecuniary gain. A study in Oslo indicated that 1.4% of pupils surveyed had sold sex. Boys were more often involved than girls. Adolescents who had sold sex were more lonely and more often reported symptoms of depression and anxiety. There was an association with conduct problems, alcohol and drug use. The majority reported no contact with any helping agency, which indicates the need for more prevention and intervention (Pederson & Hegna, 2000).

Substance use, sexual abuse and prostitution have complex cause-and-effect relationships and many common antecedent factors. In young people, common factors include poverty, homelessness, and a history of physical and emotional abuse and of psychiatric illness.

Typically, young women and men become involved in prostitution as a method of funding substance use. The source of drugs may be a pimp, a situation likely to carry the risk of violence and little direct financial reward. Homeless young people involved in the sex industry may be entrapped by older people, usually men, who initially seem protective. Many young males who have sex with men (sometimes referred to as rent boys) do not self-identify as gay and therefore are not reached by health promotion aimed at gay men. They are likely to be involved in high-risk sexual behaviour and require carefully delivered messages regarding condom use and personal protection (Rietmeijer *et al*, 1998).

The emotional and physical discomfort of sex working may be associated with escalating levels of substance use and a complex problem of affordability. Cocaine is a powerful reinforcer owing to its capacity to reduce pain and increase endurance. Alcohol and benzodiazepines (minor tranquillisers) are favoured for their effect in reducing self-awareness and recall, while heroin can numb emotional experience. One or more sedative or stimulant substances may be used to enable the cycle of stress and nocturnal wakefulness.

Sex working carries risks of sexually transmitted infections in addition to the blood-borne viruses HIV and hepatitis B and C, which are also associated with substance use. Clients of sex workers are more likely to bring additional exposure to bacterial infections (Elifson *et al*, 1999), especially gonorrhoea, syphilis and chlamydia, which carry risks of future infertility and pelvic disease. While condom use has increased among sex workers, they remain at risk of sexually transmitted infection. Studies indicate that the major risks are encountered by men and women through non-commercial partnerships rather than with clients (Ward *et al*, 1999). About a third of males who have commercial sex with men do not identify as gay and may not access relevant health information.

Violence is a significant hazard within the sex industry. Studies have shown that previous sexual assault is a factor predisposing to work in the industry and that such work carries a high risk of further assaults. In one study, 44% had had violence inflicted upon them in the previous year, while 58% had experienced rape at some time (Morrison *et al*, 1994). Psychiatric complications include depression, anxiety and post-traumatic stress disorder (Mathews *et al*, 2000). For many, these complications endure into older life (Bownes *et al*, 1991).

Studies of street prostitutes found their main needs to be protection from assaults, social support, counselling, addictions treatment and medical care (Valera *et al*, 2001).

Important interventions include outreach work, social care, screening and treatment for sexually acquired infections, treatment for substance use and, in younger people, the involvement of social services with a view to child protection. These and other related aspects are covered in Chapter 12.

Conclusion

Past experience and the later social, physical and psychological complications of substance use may interact to lead to complex social problems very quickly. Young substance misusers are vulnerable to exploitation, particularly if they are homeless, have a learning disability or are psychiatrically ill. The presence of coercive adults, sexual exploitation, parental neglect or severe behavioural problems indicates the need for services to work together in a collaborative way (Health Advisory Service, 2001). The need for formal implementation of child protection proceedings may occasionally arise. Review of this area indicates that it is imperative to view the young person's substance misuse in the context of multiple social influences and associations, each interacting with each other, which may facilitate or impair psychological and pharmacological treatment.

References

Adger, H. (1991) Problems of alcohol and other drug use and abuse in adolescents. *Journal of Adolescent Health Care*, **12**, 606–613.

Best, D., Rawaf, S., Rowley, J., *et al* (2000) Drinking and smoking as concurrent predictors of illicit drug use and positive drug attitudes in adolescents. *Drug and Alcohol Dependence*, **60**, 319–321.

Bownes, I. T., O'Gorman, E. C. & Sayer, A. (1991) Assault characteristics and posttraumatic stress disorder in victims. *Acta Psychiatrica Scandinavica*, **83**, 27–30.

Brook, D. & Brook, J. (1990) The aetiology and consequences of adolescent drug use. In *Drug and Alcohol Abuse Prevention* (ed R. Warson), pp. 339–362. Clifton, New Jersey: Humana Press.

Commander, M. J., Odell, S. O., Williams, K. S., *et al* (1999) Pathways to care for alcohol use disorders. *Journal of Public Health Medicine*, **21**, 65–69.

Crome, I. B., Christian, J. & Green, C. (2000) The development of a unique designated community drug service for adolescents: Policy, prevention and education implications. *Drugs, Education, Prevention and Policy*, **7**, 87–107.

Elifson, K. W., Boles, J., Darrow, W. W., *et al* (1999) HIV seroprevalence and risk factors among clients of female and male prostitutes. *Journal of Acquired Immune Deficiency Syndromes and Human Retrovirology*, **20**, 195–200.

Ellickson, P. L., Tucjer, J. S., Klein, D. J. O., *et al* (2001) Prospective risk factors for alcohol misuse in late adolescence. *Journal of Studies on Alcohol*, **62**, 773–782.

Emery, R., Weintraub, S. & Neale, J. M. (1982) Effects of marital discord on the school behaviour of children of schizophrenic, affectively disordered, and normal parents. *Journal of Abnormal Child Psychology*, **10**, 215–228.

Guo, J., Hawkins, J. D., Hill, K. G., *et al* (2001) Childhood and adolescent predictors of alcohol use and dependence in young adulthood. *Journal of Studies on Alcohol*, **62**, 754–762.

Health Advisory Service (2001) *The Substance of Young Needs*: London: The Home Office Drugs Prevention Advisory Service.

Kumpulainen, K. (2000) Psychiatric symptoms and deviance in early adolescence predict heavy alcohol use 3 years later. *Addiction*, **95**, 1847–1857.

Lewis, G. & Drife, J. (eds) (2002) *Why mothers die 1997–1999: The fifth report of the confidential enquiries into maternal deaths in the United Kingdom*. London: Royal College of Obstetricians and Gynaecologists.

London Health Observatory (2003) *Drug Use in London*. At http://www.lho.org.uk/hil/drug.htm

Marsden, J., Gossop, M., Stewart, D., *et al* (2000) Psychiatric symptoms among clients seeking treatment for drug dependence: Intake data from the National Treatment Outcome Research Study. *British Journal of Psychiatry*, **176**, 285–289.

Martin, S. L., Clark, K. A., Lynch, S. R., *et al* (1999) Violence in the lives of pregnant teenage women: association with multiple substance use. *American Journal of Drug and Alcohol Abuse*, **25**, 425–440.

Matthews, M., Meaden, J., Petrak, J., *et al* (2000) Psychological consequences of sexual assault among female attenders at a genitourinary medicine clinic. *Sexually Transmitted Infections*, **76**, 49–50.

McKirnan, D. J. & Peterson, P. L. (1988) Stress, expectancies, and vulnerability to substance abuse: A test of a model among homosexual men. *Journal of Abnormal Psychology*, **97**, 461–466.

Mensch, B. & Kandel, D. B. (1992) Drug use as a risk factor for premarital teen pregnancy and abortion in a national sample of young white women. *Demography*, **29**, 409–427.

Mezey, G. C. & Bewley, S. (1997) Domestic violence and pregnancy. *British Journal of Obstetrics & Gynaecology*, **104**, 528–531.

Morrison, C. L., Ruben, S. M. and Wakefield, D. (1994) Female street prostitutes in Liverpool. *AIDS*, **8**, 1194–1195.

Neale, J. (2000) Suicidal intent in non-fatal illicit drug overdose. *Addiction*, **95**, 85–93.

Nowinski, J. (1990) *Substance Abuse in Adolescents and Young Adults: A guide to treatment*. New York: Norton.

Odell, S. M., Surtees, P. G., Wainwright, N. W., *et al* (1997) Determinants of general practitioner recognition of psychological problems in a multi-ethnic inner-city health district. *British Journal of Psychiatry*, **171**, 537–541.

Office for National Statistics. (2000) *Survey of the Health and Well-being of Homeless People in Glasgow*. London: Department of Health.

Pederson, W. & Hegna, K. (2000) Children and adolescents selling sex. *Tidsskr Nor Laegeforen*, **120**, 215–220.

Rietmeijer, C. A., Wolitski, R. J., Fishbein, M., *et al* (1998) Sex hustling, injection drug use, and non-gay identification by men who have sex with men: associations with high-risk sexual behaviors and condom use. *Sexually Transmitted Diseases*, **25**, 353–360.

Rutter, M. (1985) Resilience in the face of adversity: protective factors and resilience to psychiatric disorder. *British Journal of Psychiatry*, **14**, 598–611.

Ryan, C. & Futterman, D. (1998) *Lesbian and Gay Youth, Care and Counselling*. New York: Columbia University Press.

Stoker, A. & Swadi, H. (1990) Perceived family relationships in drug abusing adolescents. *Drug and Alcohol Dependence*, **25**, 293–297.

Valera, R. J., Sawyer, R. G. & Schiraldi, G. R. (2001) Perceived health needs of inner city prostitutes: a preliminary study. *American Journal of Health Behavior*, **25**, 50–59.

Ward, H., Day, S. & Weber, J. (1999) Risky business: health and safety in the sex industry over a 9 year period. *Sexually Transmitted Infection*, **75**, 340–343.

— , Pallecaros, A., Green, A. *et al* (2000) Health issues associated with increasing use of crack cocaine among female sex workers in London. *Sexually Transmitted Infection*, **76**, 292–293.

Williams, R. & Morgan, H. (1994) *Suicide Prevention – the Challenge Confronted*. NHS London: NHS Health Advisory Service, HMSO.

CHAPTER 6

Psychiatric comorbidity

Ilana B. Crome

Key points

- There is no uniformly accepted definition of comorbidity.
- The association of psychiatric disorder with substance misuse in young people is extensively documented.
- Affective disorders, personality difficulties, eating problems and attention-deficit hyperactivity disorder are related to substance misuse.
- Substance misuse is a powerful predictor of suicide.
- Psychiatric disorders that begin in childhood have a strong likelihood of continuing into later life, and may be complicated by substance misuse as a result of the raised prevalence of the latter.
- Skilled assessment and effective treatment will help to prevent and alleviate disabling and life-threatening comorbid conditions.
- There is a need for longitudinal multi-disciplinary approaches to enhance the understanding of the patterns and severity of co-existing substance misuse and psychiatric disorder and provide pointers for novel treatments.

Introduction: the interaction between substance use and mental health

In this chapter the term 'comorbidity' is used to describe the coexistence of psychiatric disorder and substance misuse. This multiplicity of complex presentations has also been referred to as 'dual diagnosis'. This may be a confusing term, and even a misnomer, since many young people are misusing, and may even be dependent upon, multiple substances, to a varying degree and with differing psychological effects. Furthermore, both intoxication and withdrawal produce psychological symptoms.

Among young people perhaps 30–50% of those with psychiatric disorders, especially disruptive behaviour disorders, have substance misuse problems (Zeitlin, 1999). Similarly, clinical impression and the adult literature suggest that about 30–50% of substance misusers have psychiatric disorders (Crome, 1999). While much of the available data are North American, information is beginning to accumulate in Europe and the United Kingdom.

The substances that are most commonly used by young people are alcohol, nicotine and cannabis. In general, chronic use and intoxication with depressant drugs and withdrawal from stimulants produce symptoms similar to depressive disorders. Acute and chronic intoxication with stimulants or cannabis may mimic a schizophrenia-like illness. Conversely, withdrawal from depressant drugs may result in symptoms of anxiety, generalised phobic anxiety or panic disorders, as well as confusional states with psychotic features. However, it should be noted that opioids, sedatives and hypnotics, cocaine, stimulants (including caffeine), hallucinogens and volatile substances are not only related to the development of psychiatric disorder, but may even be the cause of death.

The combination of substance misuse and psychiatric disorder is associated with multiple difficulties. Drug use itself interferes with normal cognitive, emotional and social development (Fergusson & Horwood, 1997). Treatment non-compliance is reflected in missed appointments and relapse, which lead to increased hospital admissions and out-patient visits. Psychiatric illness, earlier age at onset of mood and psychotic illness and suicide attempts are also related to a poorer prognosis. Comorbidity may be reflected by poorer health in the short and longer term (e.g. poor ophthalmic and dental care, infections, epilepsy, respiratory problems, cancer and hypertension) and ultimately premature death. To compound these difficulties, this group of users frequently distances itself from professionals and is described as 'hard to engage' or 'difficult to manage' or 'vulnerable and disadvantaged'. This is displayed in their violence and aggression – as both perpetrators and victims – their homelessness and their criminal activities.

Multiple pathology has been highlighted by a study of injecting drug users. When examining poly-drug dependence and psychiatric co-morbidity among heroin injectors, Darke & Ross (1997) reported that the number of comorbid (anxiety, depression) diagnoses independently predicted the number of dependence diagnoses. In a similar study of injectors and non-injectors, the number of conduct disorder symptoms discriminated between subsequent injecting and non-injecting drug use (Neumark & Anthony, 1997). Furthermore, Milich et al (2000) have shown that while abstainers were never more psychologically impaired than experimenters, frequent users were more impaired than abstainers and experimenters.

In the light of the numerous and complex coexisting problems that this group of young people suffer, they may present at child and adolescent services, to their general practitioner, in the hospital accident and emergency department, in the paediatric department, at social services or at the educational services, but also in youth offender teams, in police stations and in residential institutions. This dispersal may lead to an underestimation of the number involved and deprive them of a coordinated assessment and specialist services.

The relationship between substance misuse and particular psychiatric disorders

Kandel *et al* (1997, 1999) studied a representative community sample of 401 adolescents (aged 14–18 years). Twenty-two per cent reported cigarette use in the previous six months, 13% (recognised as an unusually low prevalence) had used illicit drugs, and 66% had drunk alcohol in the previous year. Daily smoking, weekly alcohol consumption and use of any illicit substance in the previous year predicted both substance use disorder (i.e. substance 'abuse' or dependence) and other psychiatric disorders (anxiety, depression or disruptive behaviour). Six per cent had a diagnosis of substance use disorder and this increased with age. Furthermore, among adolescents with substance use disorder, 76% had anxiety, mood disorders or disruptive behaviour, compared with 25% of adolescents who did not. However, in this study when disruptive behaviour disorders were controlled for, the association with mood or anxiety disorder became non-significant. Although the sample with substance use disorders was small, the finding points to the hazard posed by disruptive behaviour disorder.

Depression and smoking

Escobedo *et al* (1998) analysed data from the TAPS (Teenage Attitudes and Practices Survey), a prospective cohort study of predictions of smoking (with inhalation) among US adolescents. Smoking behaviour and depressive symptoms were assessed. Adolescent females were more likely than males to report depressive symptoms and, in general, adolescent males were more likely to start to smoke. Depressed adolescents were significantly more likely than their non-depressed counterparts to start smoking. Increasing frequency of depressive symptoms was associated with graded increases in rates of smoke inhalation, suggesting a dose–response relationship. Although the difference in the rates of depressive symptoms among non-smokers (at 13%) and smokers (at 20%) was relatively small, over the population at risk this translates into large numbers of depressed adolescents who are at risk of smoking. Both depression and the development of dependence on illicit substances were related to smoking at an early age (Hanna & Grant, 1999).

A similar study was reported by Sonntag *et al* (2000). Baseline and four-year follow-up data from the Early Developmental Stages of Psychopathology (EDSP) Study on 3021 adolescents were obtained. At baseline, 36% of the sample were regular smokers and 19% were nicotine dependent. Twenty-seven per cent reported one social fear and 7% met diagnostic criteria for social phobia. Cross-sectional analysis revealed a significant association between smoking and social fears and social phobia. This was confirmed by prospective longitudinal analysis.

This is in keeping with findings by Riggs *et al* (1999), who reported that major depression was significantly associated with nicotine dependence among delinquent populations. Hence, early-onset depressive disorders, and possibly anxiety, are related to smoking and misuse of other substances.

Although the roots of use of nicotine and of other substances overlap (Fergusson *et al*, 1993, 1996), it may be that, compared with illicit substance use, the comorbid associations of smoking relate somewhat more to affective than to disruptive behavioural psychiatric disturbance. This raises the question of specific patterns of association of particular substances with specific types of psychiatric disorder.

Major depression and substance misuse

The relationship between affective disorders and substance use, in particular whether there is evidence of self-medication, poses one of the intriguing questions about comorbidity. However, few have controlled for the role of conduct disorder, that is, have examined whether, in the absence of conduct disorder, affective symptoms or disorders are still associated with substance misuse.

One exception is the study by Wilens *et al* (1999), who compared childhood-onset bipolar disorder with adolescent-onset bipolar (mania and depression) disorder and the relationship with substance use disorder. They argued that adolescent-onset bipolar disorder was strongly associated with substance use disorder, even in the absence of conduct disorder. In their opinion, adolescents with mood 'lability and dyscontrol ... self-medicate their irritable mood, aggressivity and "affective storms", as reported in adult populations' (e.g. Winokur *et al*, 1995).

In an investigation of the predictors of substance misuse in major depression, 103 adolescent in-patients with major depression were studied (King *et al*, 1996). The clinical profiles in girls that predicted substance misuse comprised longer depressive episodes, more symptoms of conduct disorder, psychosocial impairment and more active involvement in relationships with boys. For boys, conduct disorder, older age and school work problems identified depressed adolescents misusing substances. The need to identify substance misuse was highlighted, owing to the risk of self-harm related to depression and alcohol misuse.

Depression, conduct disorder and substance misuse

A treated group of 60 delinquent boys was assessed for substance use, psychiatric disorder and aggressiveness (Young *et al*, 1995). All met criteria for conduct disorder and 20% had depressive diagnoses. By age 13, nearly 80% had begun regular substance misuse: marijuana was the first substance among 42% of the group. The boys with substance dependence on average were on 3.2 different drugs, while those with 'abuse' were using, on average, one additional drug. It should be noted that conduct disorder symptoms began 3.6 years before regular use of substances. Conduct disorder symptom count and number of dependence diagnoses, but not depression, were related to suicide attempts or self-injury. More recently, Costello *et al* (1999) reported that depression and conduct disorder were associated with a higher rate and earlier onset of substance use and misuse in boys and girls.

In a longitudinal representative community study, Kumpulainen (2000) interviewed annually 1420 children aged 9, 11 and 13 years at intake. By age 16, more than half the sample had reported substance use, and 6% reported misuse or dependence. Surprisingly, anxiety predicted later onset of smoking. However, independently of conduct disorder symptoms, self- and parent-reported depression was associated with an earlier onset and a higher rate of substance misuse in both sexes. Indeed, in another study, parental ratings of disruptive behaviour were more predictive of later substance misuse than were teacher reports (Ebeling *et al*, 1999).

Using an unusual epidemiological sample of girls only, Marmorstein & Iacono (2001) reported that major depressive disorder and conduct disorder were separately associated with substance misuse and dependence. Those with both disorders demonstrated particularly high numbers of symptoms of substance misuse and dependence. The authors concluded that 'substance use problems are the norm' among girls with the combined disorder. Similarly, among young people referred for treatment of either conduct disorder or substance use disorder, the prevalence of major depression was six times higher than among non-referred controls (Crowley *et al*, 2001).

In an in-patient setting for adolescent substance misusers, 82% met a diagnosis for an axis I psychiatric disorder (Stowell & Estroff, 1992). Three-quarters of the comorbid group had two or more psychiatric disorders, of which mood disorder was most common (61%), followed by conduct disorder (54%) and anxiety disorder (43%). These results argue strongly for the simultaneous evaluation of both substance use and psychiatric disorder in this type of population.

The association between conduct disorder and substance use disorder was further explored in a sample of adolescent in-patients (Grilo *et al*, 1996). The study compared patients with conduct disorder only (*n* = 25), substance use disorder only (*n* = 24) and combined conduct disorder and substance use disorder (*n* = 54). The groups with substance use disorder only, and combined conduct disorder and substance use disorder, had borderline personality disorder more frequently than patients with conduct disorder only. (Borderline personality disorder is characterised by emotional instability that leads to explosive outbursts, transient psychotic episodes, and self-harm, including overdoses and serious suicide attempts.) Patients with conduct disorder alone had an earlier age of presentation and were diagnosed with attention-deficit hyperactivity disorder more frequently than those with combined conduct disorder and substance use disorder or substance use disorder alone. The same authors examined personality disorder in adolescent in-patients with major depression, substance use disorder, or both (Grilo *et al*, 1997). Borderline personality disorder was diagnosed more frequently in the combined group than in the mono-diagnostic groups.

Crowley *et al* (1998) scrutinised males aged 13–19 years who received residential treatment for conduct disorder and substance use disorder. At intake, assessment of these two disorders, in addition to attention-deficit hyperactivity disorder and depression, was performed; re-assessments were then made 6, 12 and 24 months later. At intake, almost all had substance use disorder and conduct disorder, with violence and criminality. Two-year follow-up revealed improvements in all comorbid conditions, but substance use remained much the same. Intake measures of the severity of substance use and conduct disorder were related to crime, conduct and substance use at two years. In summary, earlier age at onset of conduct disorder, more severe conduct disorder, and more severe dependence predicted more negative outcomes.

The finding that the rates of psychiatric disorders, particularly disruptive behaviour disorders, are much higher among adolescents with current substance use disorders than among adolescents without substance use disorders is replicated throughout the literature. However, several issues remain to be determined. These include the relationships of different disruptive behaviour disorders to substance use, the independent association of affective and anxiety disorders with substance use, and the direction of causality. In a study of young people attending a psychiatric clinic, the effect of conduct disorder on drug and alcohol use was largely mediated through facilitative peer groups (Donenberg *et al*, 2001). In the absence of the latter, conduct disorder did not predict substance use. This is consistent with the view that predisposed young people affiliate with like-minded peers, so potentiating problematic behaviour.

Deliberate self-harm and suicide

A number of studies conclude that substance misuse is a very strong predictor of suicide. There is a substantial literature on adolescent suicide completers that links psychiatric disorder, especially conduct disorder, substance misuse and completed suicide.

Renaud *et al* (1999) compared suicide completers and community controls with disruptive behaviour disorders, predominantly conduct disorder. Those who committed suicide had higher rates of current (but not lifetime) substance misuse, of past suicide attempts, of a family history of substance misuse and of mood disorder. The authors argued that since risk was attached to current rather than lifetime substance misuse, the risk was attached to 'the acute and sub-acute effects of substance abuse', possibly linked with reduction in brain serotonin, which would impair judgement and heighten impulsivity. They concluded that disruptive adolescents appear to be at substantially increased risk for completed suicide when comorbid substance misuse and a history of a suicide attempt are present. The risk increases if adolescents have a history of physical abuse, and have parents with substance misuse and mood disorders. It is possible that increasing rates of substance use, and of conduct disorder, have contributed substantially to the high rates of completed suicide in young men that prevail currently in Western societies.

Ninety-one per cent (1792) of 1969 adolescent psychiatric in-patients were traced after a mean follow-up period of 15 years (Kjelsberg *et al*, 1995). Thirty-nine had died of drug overdose. An additional 16 drug- and alcohol-related deaths had occurred. Seventy-two per cent of the 39 overdose cases had a diagnosis of opiate dependence, and the rest had poly-substance dependence. The authors compared the 39 overdose suicides with 39 surviving controls and 35 suicides from the same population. The suicide cases had more psychiatric symptoms, suicidal ideation, learning disability and somatic disorders; they also had less follow-up and were discharged on to the street and did not enter drug treatment programmes. In a later study, Kjelsberg *et al* (1999) reported that approximately 40% of those with psychoactive substance use and 'poor impulse control' ultimately died by suicide. This points to the potentially lethal mix of personality disorder and substance misuse.

Several UK studies corroborate these findings. Fombonne (1998) investigated 6091 subjects referred to psychiatric services between 1970 and 1990. Suicidal behaviours increased significantly over time among pubertal male adolescents only. The rates of suicidal behaviour and substance misuse almost doubled in this group between 1979 and 1990. The author emphasised that alcohol was the causal factor, and substance misuse predated suicidal behaviour. In a psychological autopsy, Appleby *et al* (1999) confirmed that young people committing suicide were more likely to have used alcohol or drugs, while Hawton *et al* (1999) confirmed that alcohol consumption was present in almost two-fifths of suicides in under-25-year-olds.

Psychosis and substance misuse

It is important to recognise that the substance misuser may present with psychotic symptoms due to intoxication or withdrawal. Dukes *et al* (2001) reported a census survey in which 16% of individuals with schizophrenia reported a lifetime history of non-alcohol substance misuse. Schizophrenia is relatively rare in children and young teenagers, yet half of all adults with schizophrenia have demonstrated emotional or behavioural problems before the age of 16 years (e.g. aggression, learning difficulties, unpredictable behaviour). Mostly, this constellation of behaviour will go undiagnosed as a psychotic disorder until later. However, the increasing rate of substance misuse in young people leads to the psychotic disorder being erroneously attributed to the effects of substances. In clinical practice this distinction is often difficult to make. A thorough history, corroborated by investigations and repeated contact and assessment, is usually required.

Other associated disorders

Biederman *et al* (2001) have demonstrated that, among young people with persistent attention-deficit hyperactivity disorder, there are much higher levels of substance use disorder, and alcohol, drug and nicotine dependence. However, this was substantially confined to those with persistent conduct disorder as well as attention-deficit hyperactivity disorder, compared with those with persistent attention-deficit hyperactivity disorder alone. Approximately 42% of those with persistent combined disorder showed a substance use disorder.

A Japanese study (Suzuki *et al*, 1995) established that both male and female bulimic patients exhibited more alcohol misuse than non-bulimic controls. However, only female bulimics had a higher incidence of smoking than controls. Another study (Wiederman & Pryor, 1996) investigated substance use among adolescent girls with anorexia and bulimia nervosa. Nearly one-third of girls with bulimia nervosa smoked cigarettes, had used marijuana and were drinking alcohol at least weekly, and there were increased rates of attempted suicide, stealing and sexual intercourse. Results of a study by Lipschitz *et al* (2000) indicated that post-traumatic stress symptoms and problematic substance use were associated among girls but not boys.

Effects of childhood problems in later life

A longitudinal study conducted over nine years by Brook *et al* (1998) examined the temporal relationship between psychiatric disorder and substance use disorder. A significant relationship between adolescent drug use and later depressive and disruptive disorder in young adulthood was reported.

Rowe et al (1996) examined the effect of a history of conduct disorder on major depression in 103 adults. Depressed adults with a history of conduct disorder were more likely to meet the criteria for personality disorder and had significantly higher lifetime rates of alcohol and drug dependence than those without such a history.

Mueser et al (1999) investigated the relationships between childhood conduct disorder, antisocial personality disorder and substance use disorders in psychiatric patients with severe mental illness (i.e. schizophrenia spectrum and major affective disorders). They established that childhood conduct disorder and its adult counterpart, antisocial personality disorder, represent significant risk factors for substance use disorders in severe mental illness.

Cross-sectional and prospective analysis of data on 20 291 individuals in the Epidemiologic Catchment Area (ECA) study were analysed to determine onset of anxiety, mood and addictive disorders within a one-year prospective period (Regier et al, 1998). Onset of anxiety disorder (16.4 years) and onset of social phobias (11.6 years) were some 10 years earlier than onset of major depression and panic disorder (23.2 years). This early vulnerability to anxiety and social phobias predisposed those affected to the later development of substance misuse and depression.

A longitudinal study analysed the relationship of substance misuse to later psychiatric disorder and the development of psychiatric disorder and later substance misuse (Hanna & Grant, 1999). Tobacco had the greatest impact on rates of conduct and depressive disorder, although these problems were also significantly related to level of alcohol, marijuana and other illicit drug use. Levels of adolescent tobacco and illicit drug use predicted young adult antisocial personality disorder, depression and anxiety; alcohol use predicted anxiety, and marijuana use was related to attention-deficit hyperactivity disorder.

Brown et al (1996) conducted a prospective longitudinal study of 166 adolescent boys (n = 99) and girls (n = 67), of mean age 15.9 years. Consecutive patients admitted to two adolescent addiction in-patient units were interviewed during their stay, and after six months and two years. Forty-seven per cent met the criteria for conduct disorder, which was independent of behaviours related to drug and alcohol use. Boys displayed more such behaviours, although there was a similar incidence among girls. A history of conduct disorder, independent of drug and alcohol involvement, was related to greater post-treatment alcohol use and a later diagnosis of antisocial personality disorder. Thus, while almost half of delinquent behaviours were related to drug and alcohol use, a primary diagnosis of conduct disorder was related to poorer outcome at two years.

Conclusion

Despite the fact that there is no uniformly accepted definition of comorbidity, several important themes emerge. One is the extensive documentation of the association of substance misuse with an array of psychiatric disorders (Zeitlin, 1999). Representative community samples as well as clinical samples – mostly cross-sectional, but a few longitudinal – demonstrate that a number of disorders are connected. Affective disorders (i.e. bipolar depression, major depression, anxiety, panic, phobias and post-traumatic stress syndrome) form one group. Personality problems (i.e. conduct, borderline and antisocial personality disorders) form another cluster. In addition, eating disorders and attention-deficit hyperactivity disorder are correlated with substance misuse. For some disorders, although clinical experience suggests that there is a relationship, documented reports are not available. One such example is learning disability. Most worrying of all, however, is the recurrent finding that the use of substances is strongly linked to suicide. Prevention of substance misuse is integral to suicide prevention.

A second theme relates to the recognition that psychiatric disorders that begin in childhood have a strong likelihood of continuing into later life. These conditions may be complicated by substance misuse, which is rising in prevalence and decreasing in age at onset among young people. Skilled assessment and effective treatment will help to prevent, or at least alleviate, disabling or even life-threatening comorbid conditions in young adulthood.

The need for more longitudinal multi-disciplinary approaches is the third theme. Further exploration of diagnostic classification and the development of practical assessment instruments would increase information about the patterns and severity of psychiatric disorder and the extent and type of substance misuse. This might facilitate the development of innovative treatments, which could be tested in appropriate settings. So far, this is badly lacking.

References

Appleby, L., Cooper, J., Amos, T., *et al* (1999) Psychological autopsy study of suicides by people aged under 35. *British Journal of Psychiatry*, **175**, 168–174.

Biederman, J., Mick, E., Faraone, S., *et al* (2001) Patterns of remission and symptoms decline in conduct disorder: a four year prospective study of an ADHD sample. *Journal of the American Academy of Child and Adolescent Psychiatry*, **40**, 299–306.

Brook, J. S., Cohen, P. & Brook, D. (1998) Longitudinal study of co-occurring psychiatric disorders and substance use. *Journal of the American Academy of Child and Adolescent Psychiatry*, **37**, 322–330.

Brown, S. A., Gleghorn, A., Schuckit, M. A., *et al* (1996) Conduct disorder among adolescent alcohol and drug abusers. *Journal of Studies on Alcohol*, **57**, 314–324.

Costello, E. J., Erkanli, A., Federman, E., *et al* (1999) Development of psychiatric comorbidity with substance abuse in adolescents: effects of timing and sex. *Journal of Clinical Child Psychology*, **28**, 298–311.

Crome, I. B. (1999) Substance misuse and psychiatric comorbidity: towards improved service provision. *Drugs: Education, Prevention and Policy*, **6**, 151–174.

Crowley, T., Mikulich, S., MacDonald, M., *et al* (1998) Substance-dependent, conduct-disordered adolescent males: severity of diagnosis predicts 2-year outcome. *Drug and Alcohol Dependence*, **49**, 225–237.

——, ——, Ehlers K., *et al* (2001) Validity of structured clinical evaluations in adolescents with conduct and substance problems. *Journal of the American Academy of Child and Adolescent Psychiatry*, **40**, 265–273.

Darke, S. & Ross, J. (1997) Polydrug dependence and psychiatric comorbidity among heroin injectors. *Drug and Alcohol Dependence*, **48**, 135–141.

Donenberg, G., Emerson, E., Bryant, F., *et al* (2001) Understanding AIDS-risk behavior among adolescents in psychiatric care: links to psychopathology and peer relationships. *Journal of the American Academy of Child and Adolescent Psychiatry*, **40**, 642–653.

Dukes, P. J., Pantelis, C., McPhillips, M. A., *et al* (2001) Comorbid non-alcohol substance misuse among people with schizophrenia. *British Journal of Psychiatry*, **179**, 509–513.

Ebeling, H., Moilanen, I., Linna, S. L., *et al* (1999) Smoking and drinking habits in adolescence – links with psychiatric disturbance at the age of 8 years. *European Child and Adolescent Psychiatry*, **8** (suppl. 4), 68–76.

Escobedo, L. G., Reddy, M. & Giovino, G. A. (1998) The relationship between depressive symptoms and cigarette smoking in US adolescents. *Addiction*, **93**, 433–440.

Fergusson, D. M. & Horwood, L. J. (1997) Early onset use and psychosocial adjustment in young adults. *Addiction*, **92**, 279–296.

——, Lynskey, M. T. & Horwood, L. J. (1993) Conduct problems and attention deficit disorder in middle childhood and cannabis use by age 15. *Australia and New Zealand Journal of Psychiatry*, **27**, 673–682.

——, —— & —— (1996) Alcohol misuse and juvenile offending in adolescence. *Addiction*, **91**, 483–494.

Fombonne, E. (1998) Suicidal behaviours in vulnerable adolescents. *British Journal of Psychiatry*, **173**, 154–159.

Grilo, C. M., Becker, D. F., Fehon, D. C., *et al* (1996) Conduct disorder, substance use disorders and co-existing conduct and substance use disorders in adolescent in-patients. *American Journal of Psychiatry*, **153**, S914–S920.

——, Walker, M., Becker, D., *et al* (1997) Personality disorders in adolescents with major depression, substance use disorders, and co-existing major depression and substance use disorders. *Journal of Consulting and Clinical Psychology*, **65**, 328–332.

Hanna, E. Z. & Grant, B. F. (1999) Parallels to early onset alcohol use in the relationship of early onset smoking with drug use and DSM–IV drug and depressive disorders: findings from the national longitudinal epidemiological survey. *Alcoholism: Clinical and Experimental Research*, **23**, 513–522.

Hawton, K., Houston, K. & Shepperd, R. (1999) Suicide in young people. *British Journal of Psychiatry*, **175**, 271–276.

Kandel, D. B., Johnson, J. G., Bird, H. R., *et al* (1997) Psychiatric disorders associated with substance use among children and adolescents: findings from the Methods for the Epidemiology of Child and Adolescent Mental Disorders (MECA) study. *Journal of Abnormal Child Psychology*, **25**, 121–132.

——, ——, ——, et al (1999) Psychiatric comorbidity among adolescents with substance use disorders: findings form the MECA study. *Journal of the American Academy of Child and Adolescent Psychiatry*, **38**, 693–699.

King, C. A., Guaziuddin, N., McGovern, L., et al (1996) Predictors of comorbid alcohol and substance abuse in depressed adolescents. *Journal of the American Academy of Child and Adolescent Psychiatry*, **35**, 743–751.

Kjelsberg, E., Winther, M. & Dahl, A. A. (1995) Overdose deaths in young substance abusers: accidents or hidden suicides? *Acta Psychiatrica Scandinavica*, **91**, 236–242.

——, Sandvik, L. & Dahl, A. A. (1999) A long-term follow-up study of adolescent psychiatric in-patients. Part I: Predictors of early death. *Acta Psychiatrica Scandinavica*, **99**, 231–236.

Kumpulainen, K. (2000) Psychiatric symptoms and deviance in early adolescence predict heavy alcohol use 3 years later. *Addiction*, **95**, 1847–1857.

Lipschitz, D. S., Grilo C. M., Fehon, D., et al (2000) Gender differences in the associations between post-traumatic stress symptoms and problematic substance use in psychiatric inpatient adolescents. *Journal of Mental Diseases*, **188**, 349–356.

Marmorstein, N. & Iacono, W. (2001) An investigation of female adolescent twins with both major depression and conduct disorder. *Journal of the American Academy of Child and Adolescent Psychiatry*, **40**, 299–306.

Milich, R., Lynam, D., Zimmerman, R., et al (2000) Differences in young adult psychopathology among drug abstainers, experimenters, and frequent users. *Journal of Substance Abuse*, **11**, 69–88.

Mueser, K. T., Rosenberg, S., Drake, R., et al (1999) Conduct disorder, antisocial personality disorder and substance use disorder in schizophrenia and major affective disorders. *Journal of Studies on Alcohol*, **60**, 278–284.

Neumark, Y. & Anthony, J. (1997) Childhood misbehaviour and the risk of injecting drug use. *Drug and Alcohol Dependence*, **48**, 193–197.

Regier, D. A., Rae, D. S., Narrow, W. E., et al (1998) Prevalence of anxiety disorders and their comorbidity with mood and addictive disorders. *British Journal of Psychiatry*, **173** (suppl. 34), 24–28.

Renaud, J., Brent, D. A., Birmaher, B., et al (1999) Suicide in adolescents with disruptive disorders. *Journal of American Academy of Child and Adolescent Psychiatry*, **38**, 846–851.

Riggs, P., Mikulich, S., Whitmore, E., et al (1999) Relationship of AD/HD, depression, and non-tobacco substance use disorders to nicotine dependence in substance-dependent delinquents. *Drug and Alcohol Dependence*, **54**, 195–205.

Rowe, J., Sullivan, P., Mulder, R., et al (1996) The effect of a history of conduct disorder in adult major depression. *Journal of Affective Disorders*, **37**, 51–63.

Sonntag, H., Wittchen, H. U., Hofler, M., et al (2000) Are social fears and DSM–IV anxiety disorder associated with smoking and nicotine dependence in adolescents and young adults? *European Psychiatry*, **15**, 67–74.

Stowell, R. J. & Estroff, T. (1992) Psychiatric disorders in substance abusing adolescent inpatients: a pilot study. *Journal of the American Academy of Child and Adolescent Psychiatry*, **31**, 1036–1040.

Suzuki, K., Takeda, A. & Matsushita, S. (1995) Co-prevalence of bulimia and alcohol abuse and smoking among Japanese male and female high school students. *Addiction*, **90**, 971–975.

Wiederman, M. W. & Pryor, T. (1996) Substance use and impulsive behaviours among adolescents with eating disorders. *Addictive Behaviours*, **21**, 269–272.

Wilens, T., Biederman, J., Millstein, R., et al (1999) Risk of substance use disorders in youths with child and adolescent onset bipolar disorder. *Journal of the American Academy of Child and Adolescent Psychiatry*, **38**, 680–685.

Winokur, G., Coryell, W., Akiskal, H., *et al* (1995) Alcoholism in manic depressive (bipolar) illness: familial illness, course of illness and the primary–secondary distinction. *American Journal of Psychiatry*, **152**, 365–372.

Young, S. E., Mikulich, S. K., Goodwin, M. B., *et al* (1995) Treated delinquent boys: substance use onset pattern relationship to conduct and mood disorders. *Drug and Alcohol Dependence*, **37**, 149–162.

Zeitlin, H. (1999) Psychiatric comorbidity with substance misuse in children and teenagers. *Drug and Alcohol Dependence*, **55**, 225–234.

CHAPTER 7

Implications of parental substance misuse

Eilish Gilvarry and Ilana B. Crome

Key points

- In the UK, it is estimated that approximately 1 in 11 children are living in a family where alcohol is a problem and that, on average, each problematic drug user has a child.
- The impact of parental substance misuse will vary with the age and developmental stage of the child.
- There is some evidence that children of substance misusers are overrepresented in the social and health services.
- Substance misuse by parents is probably related to an increased likelihood of psychiatric, behavioural, developmental and substance misuse disorders in their children, but the evidence is not conclusive.
- There is a need to provide comprehensive and accessible services for parents and children, by involving substance misuse services with children's services at an early stage in the treatment plan when a substance-misusing parent is identified.
- Acknowledgement of the need for long-term commitment and collaborative working in terms of monitoring the whole family improves treatment outcome.

Introduction

It is important to recognise the nature and extent of substance misuse in the adult population. While approximately one-quarter of adults are drinking above the recommended 'safe limits' of four units per day for men and three units per day for adult women, this degree of excessive drinking may be found in 40% or more of the population aged 16–24 years. Five per cent of the adult population are dependent on alcohol. A quarter of the adult population are addicted to nicotine, and in young women the prevalence is increasing. Drug misuse occurs in approximately 1–2% of the adult population, but predominantly in the younger age groups. Regular cannabis use occurs in about 10% of young people.

Accurate estimates of the number of children affected by parental substance misuse are difficult to obtain. One in eight Americans is the child of an alcoholic parent (Weinberg, 1997), one in four children in the USA is exposed to family alcohol misuse or dependence (Grant, 2000) and approximately 5% of infants born each year are prenatally exposed to illicit drugs. In the UK, approximately 1 million, or one in 11, children live in a family with alcohol problems (Alcohol Concern, 2001). It is estimated that, on average, each problematic drug user in the UK has a child (Advisory Council on the Misuse of Drugs, 2003).

When young people misuse substances (and the prevalence of this is increasing, as discussed in earlier chapters), the transition to adult roles, notably parenthood, may occur precociously (Fergusson & Horwood, 1997, 2000; Fergusson et al, 2002). The potential impact of very young, often deprived, substance-misusing parents on the health and development of children requires serious consideration. This was starkly stressed in Why Mothers Die, the fifth confidential enquiry into maternal deaths (Lewis & Drife, 2001).

Children may be affected by parental substance misuse in many different ways. Exposure in utero and genetic factors may produce and interact with mental ill health, as well as physical and behavioural difficulties in both parent and child. These, in turn, are likely to result in family dysfunction. The impact of parental substance misuse will vary according to the age and developmental stage of the child. As described in Chapter 4, there is heightened awareness of the risk factors and pathways that lead to dysfunctional behaviour. Risks can be mitigated by protective factors such as consistent and caring regular monitoring by adults, attendance at school with vigilant teachers, involvement in organised after-school activities, and alternative safe accommodation if subjected to violence or the threat of violence (Cleaver et al, 1999).

Although some authorities have observed that the majority of children who grow up in alcohol- and drug-using families will not have long-term developmental or emotional sequelae and 'emerge relatively intact psychologically and emotionally' (Searles & Windle, 1990; Abel & Hannigan, 1996; Hogan, 1998), there is evidence that these children are overrepresented in social, mental and physical health services. While it is not possible to determine the precise effect on an individual child, these children generally are more susceptible than other children to injury, mental illness and substance use, which is reflected in more admissions to psychiatric units, longer lengths of stay and greater total health care costs. Increased physical problems, more frequent visits to medical out-patient departments, mainly with somatic complaints of headaches and sleep disturbance, especially in older children, are linked to parental alcohol problems (West & Prinz, 1987).

An American report illustrates significant negative effects of alcohol and drug misuse in the child welfare system (National Center on Addiction and Substance Abuse, 1999). The report noted a doubling of the numbers of abused children, which was related to drug and alcohol misuse, in the decade 1986–97. Children of substance-misusing parents are at least three times more likely to be abused or neglected. Moreover, children exposed prenatally to illicit drugs are two to three times more likely to be abused and neglected. Over 80% of child welfare professionals cited alcohol in combination with other drugs as the leading substance of misuse in child abuse and neglect cases. The report recognised that parental substance misuse is usually clustered with other problems, such as poverty, mental illness, unemployment, social isolation and past history of abuse. Likewise, in the UK, alcohol misuse was found among one-third to two-thirds of households reporting child abuse or neglect. This was associated with a greater incidence of violence and parental mental illness (Cleaver et al, 1999).

Data from child protection studies in the UK reiterate the link between child abuse and neglect and parental alcohol and drug use. The relationship with parental problems increases with the seriousness of the enquiry. In the early stages of child protection referral and first enquiry, 20–25% of parents were found to have a history of alcohol or drug problems (National Society for the Prevention of Cruelty to Children, 1997a). This rose to 25–60% at the child protection case conference stage, and to 70% if court orders were made (Rickford, 1996; Brisby et al, 1997). Kearney et al (2000) reported estimates that 50–90% of social care case-loads involve alcohol and drug problems or mental health problems. Twenty-three per cent of child neglect cases identified via helplines involve parental alcohol misuse. Parental alcohol misuse was reported in 13% of calls about emotional abuse, 10% of calls about physical abuse and 5% of calls about sexual abuse (National Society for the Prevention of Cruelty to Children, 1997b).

This represents the tip of the iceberg, since the problems range in severity and may be subtle and difficult to detect. Parents may avoid seeking help for fear that they may be separated from their children. In order to support and enhance the family and to reduce harm, it is imperative that they are identified.

Pregnancy

A combination of risk behaviours in adolescents – such as smoking, drug and alcohol misuse, delinquency and precocious sexual activities – may lead to pregnancy. These risks make engagement with services problematic for young pregnant misusers, who may be ambivalent about the pregnancy, be vulnerable to domestic violence, have comorbid psychiatric conditions, and already have a history of involvement with social services.

Research on the prevalence of substance misuse in pregnancy, the effectiveness of treatments during pregnancy and after delivery, and the impact of substance problems on the development of the foetus and child is limited (Hill *et al*, 2000). With the exception of a few studies, those that have been undertaken have had small samples and short follow-up periods. The main focus has been on tobacco, alcohol, marijuana and opiates.

Morbidity and mortality

Adolescents, particularly those under 15 years, are at higher risk for the complications of pregnancy, and have a higher death rate (Scholl *et al*, 1994). Also, mothers who smoke during pregnancy are at higher risk of mortality from respiratory and cardiovascular complications, cancer, accidents and suicides (Rantakallio *et al*, 1995). Maternal substance misuse also places the foetus at increased risk of complications such as low birth weight from nicotine and cannabis, withdrawal symptoms from heroin, methadone and cocaine, rupture of the placenta from cocaine, and foetal alcohol syndrome.

Prenatal alcohol use is the leading preventable cause of birth defects, mental retardation and neurodevelopmental disorders. Half of all pregnant women surveyed reported consuming some alcohol during the 3 months prior to pregnancy recognition (Floyd et al, 1999), 14–20% reported drinking some alcohol during the pregnancy, with 0.2–1% meeting criteria for heavy drinking (Morse & Hutchins, 2000). In the USA, the incidence of children affected by prenatal alcohol exposure ranges from 0.5 to 3.0 births per 1000, although the overall rate in the Western world has been estimated at 0.33 per 1000 live births (Abel & Sokol, 1991). In addition to the full syndrome, there are 3–5 children per 1000 who will exhibit less severe effects, termed alcohol-related birth defects. Lemoine *et al* (1968) and Jones & Smith (1973) described the dysmorphic features, growth retardation and central nervous system (CNS) problems associated with foetal alcohol syndrome. Dysmorphic features include microcephaly, micro-ophthalmia, thin upper lip and a flattening of the mid-face. CNS effects include mental retardation, hyperactivity and attention deficits, poor impulse control, and language and motor development delays (Young, 1997). Affected children continue to manifest developmental disabilities, psychiatric disorders and cognitive delay as they mature. In terms of dysmorphic features, those who were more severely damaged also showed the more prevalent and marked psychiatric symptoms. Milder difficulties in mothers drinking more than 250 g (8–10 g is one unit) of alcohol per week were noted, such as poor attention span, distractibility, and poorer performance on IQ and neurobehavioural tests. Streissguth *et al* (1994*a*,*b*), in a 14-year follow-up study, identified dose–response effects of alcohol prenatally on neurobehavioural attention, speed of information processing and learning function at age 14. Adolescent sequelae of deficits observed earlier in development were confirmed. It is estimated that six standard units of alcohol (48–60 g) can cause foetal alcohol syndrome, but low levels (e.g. 10 g per day) have not been demonstrated to produce adverse outcomes (James *et al*, 1995). Women should be discouraged from drinking more than one unit per day.

Exposure to nicotine during pregnancy results in low birth weight and intra-uterine growth restriction associated with developmental delay. A recurring theme is the association between maternal smoking during pregnancy and sudden infant death syndrome (Bauer, 1999), and the correlation of passive smoking with respiratory difficulties in infants. Duration of smoking, exposure to environmental smoke (e.g. smoking in partners and family), self-efficacy and educational methods have been shown to influence the mother's reduction in nicotine use during and after pregnancy (Woodby *et al*, 1999).

A classic opiate abstinence withdrawal syndrome occurs in at least 50% of babies born to opiate-using mothers. No clear teratogenic effect has been identified, although consistent findings include low birth weight, prematurity and reduced intra-uterine growth (Bauer, 1999). Cannabis exposure is related to shorter gestation and low birth weight, and later effects on the CNS, cognitive development and behaviour (Scher *et al*, 1988; Martin & Hall, 1998; Fergusson *et al*, 2002). A mild withdrawal syndrome has been reported, and disturbed sleep with potentiation of the effects of alcohol on the foetus have been described in relation to maternal cannabis use (Fried, 1991; Dahl *et al*, 1995). Although 'crack babies' have attracted attention in the popular press, no consistent constellation of findings in the developmental outcome of those prenatally exposed to cocaine when compared with matched controls has emerged. Maternal cocaine use in the third trimester is associated with restricted intra-uterine brain growth (Bauer, 1999; Bateman & Chiriboga, 2000). Cognitive effects appear to be related to environmental risk, social status and exposure to multiple and cumulative risks, which compromise outcomes and which may over-shadow any prenatal effect of cocaine (Tronick & Beeghly, 1999). It should also be noted that ecstasy is associated with congenital cardiovascular and musculoskeletal abnormalities (McElhatton *et al*, 1999). Prenatal exposure to any drug should be seen as a possible marker for multiple medical and social risk factors, for example social isolation, maternal psychopathology and child abuse.

Management of pregnancy

Pregnancy offers a window of opportunity for the treatment of substance problems because pharmacological, behavioural and social interventions can routinely be offered during pregnancy. If this does not take place, it may partly be related to inadequacy of screening, a lack of in-depth assessment and care planning, and the absence of coordinated services. However, it may also be related to parental concerns about the health of the baby, sensitivities about parenting ability, and inability to access proper care.

If a young pregnant substance user presents to services, the principle is synchronisation of the care package. It is helpful to have local protocols in place that routinely involve practitioners from obstetric, substance misuse and primary care services (e.g. community midwife, health visitor, general practitioner), and from paediatric, psychiatric and social services if required.

The substance misuse and the psychiatric, obstetric and medical assessment are basic issues to be addressed. Treatment during pregnancy, during labour and after delivery should be discussed, carefully planned and harmonised if there is time. Young pregnant users may present late in pregnancy, or occasionally at delivery. Drug and alcohol withdrawal (especially if there are obstetric emergencies), substitute prescribing, the type of analgesia to be used during labour, the mother's viral status and views about delivery are some issues that need to be addressed. Thereafter, breast-feeding, probable adjustment of medication, immunisation, contraception and arrangements for discharge and follow-up needs review, particularly if the baby has been in the special care baby unit, or if there are child protection issues.

Outcome in pregnancy

There is a paucity of well-controlled trials of interventions for pregnant young women who misuse substances.

One randomised trial aimed to reduce the level of drinking during pregnancy; it compared a brief intervention and comprehensive assessment to assessment only, and found reductions in drinking in both groups antenatally. However, women who were abstinent before assessment, and who received the brief intervention, maintained higher rates of abstinence during the pregnancy than the control group (Chang *et al*, 1999). Alcohol consumption has been shown to decrease during pregnancy in any event (Ihlen *et al*, 1994), so that any treatment effects need to be evaluated against this background.

Randomised controlled trials of nicotine replacement therapy for pregnant smokers are required. Given the adverse consequences of smoking for the mother and foetus, it is sensible to consider the use of nicotine replacement if there is no response to behavioural interventions (Wisborg *et al*, 2000). Indeed, recent guidance from the National Institute for Clinical Excellence (NICE) (2002) has recommended that under-18s and pregnant and breast-feeding women should be prescribed nicotine replacement therapy.

Methadone treatment as part of a comprehensive package of care for pregnant heroin users has been shown to improve birth outcomes and maternal psychosocial function (Batey & Weissel, 1993). There are problems related to the development of a prolonged neonatal methadone withdrawal syndrome, which occurs in more than 60% of infants and which may lengthen hospitalisation. For this reason, the use of buprenorphine has been explored and found to be safe and effective in the mother, foetus and infant from conception onwards. It has a further advantage that, in the UK, it is licensed for use in the 16–18-year age group (Fischer, 2000; Fischer *et al*, 2000; Schindler *et al*, 2003).

Until systematic controlled studies are undertaken, clinical decisions have to be made as to whether the potential benefits from pharmacological treatments outweigh the risks associated with continued substance misuse during pregnancy. Psychosocial interventions remain the mainstay.

Family functioning

Alcohol problems can have effects on family functioning, behaviour, and mental and physical health. Alcoholic families are characterised by increased conflict, more hostile communications and lower levels of cohesion (Von Knorring, 1991). Child-rearing practices can be rejecting, harsh and neglecting. Although anecdotal clinical reports have suggested that children of alcoholics are 'victims' of an alcoholic family environment characterised by disruption, parental role deviancy and disturbed parent–child relationships, research has demonstrated that these family patterns are not unique to those with alcohol problems.

Violence, child abuse, family separation and divorces are associated with alcohol problems. Children of drinking parents report more involvement in family arguments (Velleman & Orford, 1999). The increased family conflict may cause children to blame themselves for the drink problem, and will disturb communication, alter roles and responsibilities, and disrupt family social life (Brisby *et al*, 1997; Houston *et al*, 1997; Velleman & Orford, 1999).

Research in this area has mostly centred on the parenting styles of mothers attending drug treatment facilities or in receipt of child welfare services. Therefore it is difficult to extrapolate findings to those drug users not in treatment, or to paternal drug use. It is more likely that those attending treatment will have comorbid disorders and experience more psychological distress, although Burns *et al* (1996) reported that attendance for treatment indicated greater stability. Failure to include appropriately matched controls in much of the research makes any conclusion regarding a direct causal association between family functioning or parenting styles with drug use unconvincing.

Hogan (1998) has suggested that the experiences of children brought up in families of those who use drugs are different from those of children in the care of those who exclusively use alcohol. Drug use, to which children may be exposed at a very early age, may be perceived as more stigmatising than alcohol use. The physical environment may be dangerous as a result of intoxication or unsafe injecting equipment. Criminal activities associated with the use of illicit drugs may lead to violence or to separation due to custodial sentences. A considerable amount of time and money are spent accessing drugs. This chaotic lifestyle results in inadequate supervision, lack of routines, unstable accommodation, financial difficulties, multiple episodes of substitute care giving within and outside the family, and disrupted schooling.

Substance misuse in children of substance-misusing parents

The high risk of development of alcoholism in the children of alcoholic parents is the most robust finding from the literature (Sher, 1997). Sher reported that these children had a 2–10 times greater risk of developing alcoholism than had other children, and were at increased risk of other substance misuse and dependence, including nicotine, although the evidence was not as extensive. Weinberg (1997) similarly reported that the children of parental alcohol users are at greater risk of earlier onset of alcohol use, problematic drinking at younger ages, and heavier alcohol use than their peers, and at greater risk for other substance misuse. Difficulties in transition from adolescence to adulthood, in making friendships, in separation from home, and in peer relationships, as well as substance misuse, occur (Velleman & Orford, 1999).

There is evidence that problem drug use in parents is associated with drug use in their children (Gfroerer, 1987; Hoffman & Su, 1998). This may be related to a range of interacting factors, such as genetic factors, constitutional factors, parental attitudes and parental substance misuse. Wilens *et al* (1995) noted that children of those mothers maintained on methadone had increased rates of behavioural problems. The factors indicative of this increased risk, such as family conflict and affiliation with like-minded peers, interact to create a development process that further escalates problem behaviours.

Prenatal exposure to smoking is related to antisocial and criminal behaviour in men and drug use in women (Brennan *et al*, 1999). The research evidence, although seriously flawed, suggests that the children of drug users may be at more risk of neglect. However, complicating factors include the high prevalence of coexisting mental health problems, and there is some evidence that comorbid disorders may be associated with more parenting difficulties in drug users than in non-drug users (Mayes, 1995).

Psychiatric and behavioural difficulties in children of substance-misusing parents

Alcohol

Most studies report associations between mental health problems and parental drinking. Teenagers of parents who misuse alcohol may be at greater risk of: psychiatric problems (e.g. mood and anxiety disorders); substance problems (i.e. substance use and dependence); and behavioural problems (e.g. conduct disorder, aggression, temper tantrums, truancy and delinquency) (Connolly *et al*, 1993; Lynskey *et al*, 1994; Steinhausen, 1995). Lynskey *et al* (1994) reported that the prevalence of these disorders was between 2.2 and 3.9 times higher in the offspring of parental alcohol misusers than in those without parental alcohol problems. A 12-year follow-up study demonstrated a correlation between length of prenatal alcohol exposure and behavioural problems (Autti-Ramo, 2000). Maternal alcohol problems appear to be related to depression in offspring, especially females (Chassin *et al*, 2000; O'Connor & Kasari, 2000).

Because of the impulsivity, hyperactivity, poor self-control and impairment in concentration often described in the children of alcoholic parents, many studies report the association of attention-deficit hyperactivity disorder with parental alcohol misuse, but this is not conclusive (Reich *et al*, 1993). Despite the apparently strong association between parental drinking and emotional and behavioural disorders in children (Reich *et al*, 1993), most of the research is descriptive and it is difficult to attribute any direct causal link to alcohol. Environmental factors such as parental comorbidity and family disharmony, as well as genetic factors, may have confounding effects on the development of these disorders.

Sher (1997) investigated whether specific personality traits character-ise the adult children of parents with alcohol problems and concluded that impulsivity and disinhibition did so, although the magnitude of the effect was small. He cautioned against making generalisations about the psychological problems of these children from the available literature, although the increased risk was acknowledged.

Drugs

The children of people who use narcotics appear to be at high risk of developing substance misuse and other deviant behaviours (Nurco *et al*, 1999). Nunes *et al* (1998) noted that sons of opiate addicts with major depression were more at risk of conduct disorder, as well as social and intellectual impairment, when compared with sons of opiate users without depression and controls. Nunes *et al* postulated that the predominant psychopathology, drug dependence, had been successfully treated with methadone maintenance with accompanying improvement in family functioning, and that this explained the relative lack of impairment in those children of addicts without depression. In addition, exposure to cannabis in the first and third trimesters is related to hyperactivity, inattention and impulsivity at ten years of age (Goldschmidt *et al*, 2000).

While negative effects of maternal drug use on cognitive development appear to be related to both the prenatal and the postnatal environment, the latter is probably predominant (Hogan, 1998). Children of alcoholic parents have poorer academic performance, more frequent signs of stress, behavioural problems and adjustment difficulties in school, are more often considered by teachers to have problems, are referred more frequently to school psychologists, change school more often, and also demonstrate less verbal proficiency, abstraction and conceptual reasoning (Velleman & Orford, 1999). Thus, although many studies report educational difficulties, whether these are directly attributable to neuropsychological deficits, or to a combination of behavioural difficulties and environmental factors (e.g. lack of routines and absences from school), has not been disentangled.

Genetic predisposition

Many parents who seek help for their substance use are worried that their problems may be inherited by their children. Substance use tends to run in families, and twin and adoption studies support the view that there is a genetic predisposition, or vulnerability due to genetic factors, to develop substance problems or dependence (Merikangas *et al*, 1994; Cadoret *et al*, 1995; Kendler *et al*, 1995, 1997). However, this susceptibility interacts with environmental influences, such as the availability of substances, which can exert considerable pressures on young people to initiate and continue substance misuse. Parents need to appreciate, and be reassured, that despite the fact that there is a genetic component to the development of substance problems, this does not justify therapeutic nihilism.

Of pertinence is a growing body of evidence from so-called 'high risk' or 'family history positive' studies, which demonstrates differences in biological markers in children of substance misusers compared with controls, before initiation into substance use. The studies include genetically mediated electrophysiological (EEG) and amplitude of the P300 component of event-related potential (ERP) measures, which have been shown to vary systematically in high-risk compared with low-risk individuals. Alcohol challenge studies demonstrate decreased reactions to alcohol (e.g. body sway, hormonal responses, and sensitivity to the rewarding and anxiolytic effects) in the high-risk group (Hill, 2000; Lieberman, 2000; Schuckit, 2000; Schuckit & Smith, 2001). Personality traits (e.g. novelty seeking) predict early onset of alcohol misuse, criminality and other substance misuse, and discriminate those with antisocial personality disorder from controls (Howard *et al*, 1997). Studies of neurotransmitters such as endogenous opioids, dopamine, GABA and serotonin have indicated that, for example, dopamine transmission is associated with substance misuse and the related traits of novelty seeking and attention deficit disorder.

Rapid advances in the field of genetics, such as the mapping of the entire human genome, coupled with sophisticated neuroimaging techniques, are likely to produce a greater understanding of the nature and extent of the contribution of genetic factors to the development of substance misuse and, ultimately, to improve treatments (Hill, 2000; Working Party of the Royal College of Psychiatrists and the Royal College of Physicians, 2000; Munafo *et al*, 2001).

Service delivery, policy and research directions

The Scottish Executive (2001) reported on the need for careful assessments, for protocols on information sharing between agencies, and for the provision of comprehensive accessible services for parents and children, by linking substance misuse services with children's services. This implies a need for improved multi-agency responses and relationships at policy, agency and individual levels (National Center on Addiction and Substance Abuse, 1999). In this way, timely access to services, strategies to engage children, the family and carers, and strategies to provide best practice can be enhanced. This organisational framework would acknowledge both that substance misuse is a chronic, relapsing disorder that is likely to require long-term involvement, and that there is a need to treat and monitor the whole family in terms of the substance use, parenting capacity and skills, and the development of the children. Indeed, the evidence suggests that retention in treatment is associated with improved outcomes (Hankin *et al*, 2000). It should be stressed that while many services focus on infants or younger children, many older children who are also at great risk of early initiation into substance misuse are living in substance-misusing families. Similarly, much research focuses on prenatal effects and early

95

infant development rather than on later psychosocial and cognitive development. Much more research is needed on the resilience of children who manage to cope positively with adverse circumstances (Cleaver *et al*, 1999; Velleman & Orford, 1999).

Conclusions

Several fundamental conclusions emerge. A history of parental, and even grand-parental, substance misuse must be assessed in any young substance misuser presenting for treatment. There should be a high index of suspicion regarding the possibility of substance misuse, psychiatric, behavioural, cognitive and physical difficulties in the children of any parent presenting for treatment for substance misuse. Young substance misusers must be asked whether they or their partners may be pregnant. Further in-depth assessment, advice and treatment should be planned within the context of the family background and social network. The relationship of physical, psychiatric and substance problems to presenting complaints should be carefully analysed so that a multi-faceted approach to treatment can be organised, for poverty and violence mar the lives of this group of young people (Martin *et al*, 1999). Despite the fact that there is a dearth of evidence regarding outcome for the children of young substance misusers who are both patients and parents, the results of inaction should be weighed against the advantage of good practice (Barnard, 1994; Howell *et al*, 1999) and some preliminary evidence of cost-effectiveness (Svikis *et al*, 1997).

References

Abel, E. L. & Hannigan, H. (1996) Risk factors and pathogenesis. In *Alcohol, Pregnancy and the Developing Child* (eds H. Spohr & H. Steinhausen), pp. 63–98. Cambridge: Cambridge University Press.
—— & Sokol, R. (1991) A revised conservative estimate of the incidence of foetal alcohol syndrome and its economic impact. *Alcoholism: Clinical and Experimental Research*, **15**, 514–524.
Advisory Council on the Misuse of Drugs (2003) *Hidden Harm*. London: Home Office.
Alcohol Concern (2001) Alcohol and the family: putting the children first. *Information Bulletin*, June, 1–14.
Autti-Ramo, I. (2000) Twelve year follow up of children exposed to alcohol in utero. *Developmental Medicine and Child Neurology*, **42**, 406–411.
Barnard, M. (1994) Editorial. Forbidden questions: drug dependent parents and the welfare of their children. *Addiction*, **94**, 1109–1111.
Bateman, D. A. & Chiriboga, C. A. (2000) Dose response effect of cocaine on newborn head circumference. *Pediatrics*, **106**, 33–39.
Batey, R. G. & Weissel, K. (1993) A 40 month follow up of pregnant drug using women treated at Westmead Hospital. *Drug and Alcohol Review*, **12**, 265–270.
Bauer, C. (1999) Perinatal effects of prenatal drug exposure. *Clinics in Perinatology*, **26**, 87–106.

Brennan, P. A., Grekin, E. R. & Mednick, S. A. (1999) Maternal smoking during pregnancy and adult male criminal outcomes. *Archives of General Psychiatry*, **56**, 215–219.

Brisby, T., Baker, S. & Hedderwick, T. (1997) *Under the Influence: Coping with Parents Who Drink Too Much*. London: Alcohol Concern.

Burns, E., O'Driscoll, M. & Watson, G. (1996) The health and development of children whose mothers are on methadone maintenance. *Child Abuse Review*, **5**, 113–122.

Cadoret, R. J., Yates, W. R., Troughton, E., *et al* (1995) Adoption study demonstrating two genetic pathways to drug abuse. *Archives of General Psychiatry*, **41**, 983–989.

Chang, G., Wilkins-Haug, L., Berman, S. A., *et al* (1999) Brief intervention for alcohol use in pregnancy: a randomised trial. *Addiction*, **94**, 1499–1508.

Chassin, L., Pitts, S. C., DeLucian, C., *et al* (2000) A longitudinal study of children of alcoholics: predicting young adult substance use disorders, anxiety and depression. *Journal of Abnormal Psychology*, **108**, 106–119.

Cleaver, H., Unell, I. & Aldgate, J. (1999) *Children's Needs – Parenting Capacity: The Impact of Parental Mental Illness, Problem Alcohol and Drug Use, and Domestic Violence on Children's Development*. London: Department of Health, The Stationery Office.

Connolly, G., Caswell, S., Stewart, J., *et al* (1993) The effects of parents' alcohol problems on children's behaviour as reported by parents and by teachers. *Addiction*, **88**, 1283–1290.

Dahl, R. E., Scher, M. S. & Williamson, D. (1995) A longitudinal study of prenatal marijuana use: effects on sleep and arousal at age 3 years. *Archives of Pediatric Medicine*, **149**, 145–150.

Fergusson, D. M. & Horwood, L. J. (1997) Early onset cannabis use and psychosocial adjustment in young adults. *Addiction*, **92**, 279–296.

—— & —— (2000) Does cannabis use encourage other forms of illicit drug use? *Addiction*, **95**, 505–520.

——, Horwood, L. J., Northstone, K. & the ALSPAC study team (2002) Maternal use of cannabis and pregnancy outcome. *British Journal of Obstetrics and Gynaecology*, **109**, 21–27.

Fischer, G. (2000) Treatment of opioid dependence in pregnant women. *Addiction*, **95**, 1141–1144.

——, Johnstone, R. E., Eder, H. *et al* (2000) Treatment of opioid dependent pregnant women with buprenorphine. *Addiction*, **95**, 239–244.

Floyd, R. L., Decoufle, P. & Hungerford, D. W. (1999) Alcohol use prior to pregnancy recognition. *American Journal of Preventive Medicine*, **17**, 101–107.

Fried, P. A. (1991) Marijuana use during pregnancy: consequences for the offspring. *Seminars in Perinatology*, **15**, 280–287.

Gfroerer, J. (1987) Correlation between drug use by teenagers and drug use by older family members. *American Journal of Drug and Alcohol Abuse*, **13**, 95–108.

Goldschmidt, L., Day, N. L. & Richardson, G. A. (2000) Effects of pre-natal marijuana exposure on child behaviour problems at age 10. *Neurotoxicology and Teratology*, **22**, 325–336.

Grant, B. F. (2000) Estimates of children exposed to alcohol abuse and dependence in the family. *American Journal of Public Health*, **90**, 112–115.

Hankin, J., McCaul, M. E. & Heussner, J. (2000) Pregnant alcohol abusing women. *Alcohol Clinical and Experimental Research*, **24**, 1276–1286.

Hill, S. Y. (2000) Biological phenotypes associated with individuals at high risk for developing alcohol related disorders: Part I. *Addiction Biology*, **5**, 5–22.

——, Lowers, L., Locke-Wellman, J., *et al* (2000) Maternal smoking and drinking during pregnancy and the risk for child and adolescent psychiatric disorders. *Journal of Studies on Alcohol*, **61**, 661–668.

Hoffman, J. & Su, S. S. (1998) Parental substance use disorder, mediating variables and adolescent drug use: a non recursive model. *Addiction*, **93**, 1351–1364.

Hogan, D. (1998) Annotation. The psychological development and welfare of children of opiate and cocaine users: review and research needs. *Journal of Child Psychology and Psychiatry*, **39**, 609–620.

Houston, A., Kork, S. & MacLeod, M. (1997) *Beyond the Limit: Children Who Live with Parental Alcohol Misuse*. At www.childline.org.uk.

Howard, M. O., Kivlahan, D. & Walker, R. D. (1997) Cloninger's tridimensional theory of personality and psychopathology: applications to substance use disorders. *Journal of Studies on Alcohol*, **58**, 48–66.

Howell, E. M., Heiser, N. & Harrington, M. (1999) A review of findings on substance abuse treatment for pregnant women. *Journal of Substance Abuse Treatment*, **16**, 195–219.

Ihlen, B. M., Amundsen, A., Tronnes, L., *et al* (1994) Changes in alcohol and tobacco use during pregnancy. *Nordisk Alkoholtidskrift*, **11**, 91–99.

James, D., Greenwood, R., McCabe, R., *et al* (1995) Alcohol consumption during pregnancy in Bristol. *Journal of Obstetrics and Gynaecology*, **15**, 84–87.

Jones, K. & Smith, D. (1973) Recognition of the fetal alcohol syndrome in early infancy. *Lancet*, **ii**, 999–1001.

Kearney, K., Levin, E. & Rosen, G. (2000) *Alcohol, Drug and Mental Health Problems: Working with Families*. London: National Institute for Social Work.

Kendler, K. S., Walters, E. E., Neale, M. C., *et al* (1995) The structure of the genetic and environmental risk factors for six major psychiatric disorders in women: phobia, generalised anxiety disorder, panic disorder, bulimia, major depression and alcoholism. *Archives of General Psychiatry*, **52**, 374–383.

——, Davis, C. G. & Kessler, R. C. (1997) The familial aggregation of common psychiatric and substance use disorders in the National Comorbidity Survey: a family history study. *British Journal of Psychiatry*, **170**, 541–549.

Lemoine, P., Harousseau, H., Borteyru, J., *et al* (1968) Les enfants de parents alcoholiques. Anomalies observées: à propos de 127 cas. *Quest Médical*, **21**, 476–492.

Lewis, G. & Drife, J. O. (eds) (2001) *Why Mothers Die 1997–1999: The Fifth Report of the Confidential Enquiries into Maternal Deaths in the United Kingdom*. London: Royal College of Obstetricians and Gynaecologists.

Lieberman, D. (2000) Children of alcoholics: an update. *Current Opinion in Paediatrics*, **12**, 336–340.

Lynskey, M. T., Fergusson, D. M. & Horwood, L. (1994) The effect of parental alcohol problems on rates of adolescent psychiatric disorders. *Addiction*, **89**, 1277–1286.

Martin, B. R. & Hall, A. W. (1998) The health effects of cannabis: key issues of policy relevance. *Bulletin of Narcotics*, **49–50**, 85–90.

Martin, S. L., Clark, K. A., Lynch, S. R., *et al* (1999) Violence in the lives of pregnant teenage women is associated with multiple substance use. *American Journal of Drugs and Alcohol Abuse*, **25**, 425–440.

Mayes, L. (1995) Substance abuse and parenting. In *Handbook of Parenting* (ed. M. Bornstein), pp. 101–125. Mahwah, NJ: Lawrence Erlbaum.

McElhatton, P. R., Bateman, D. N., Evans, C. *et al* (1999) Congential anomalies after prenatal ecstasy exposure. *Lancet*, **354**, 1441–1442.

Merikangas, K. R., Risch, N. J. & Wiessman, M. M. (1994) Comorbidity and co-transmission of alcoholism, anxiety and depression. *Psychological Medicine*, **24**, 69–80.

Morse, B. A. & Hutchins, E. (2000) Reducing complications from alcohol use through screening. *Journal of the American Women's Association*, **55**, 225–227.

Munafo, M., Johnstone, E., Murphy, M., *et al* (2001) New directions in the genetic mechanisms underlying nicotine addiction. *Addiction Biology*, **6**, 109–117.

National Center on Addiction and Substance Abuse (1999) *No Safe Haven: Children of Substance-Abusing Parents*. At http://www.casacolumbia.org/publications1456/publications_show.htm?doc_id=7167

National Institute for Clinical Excellence (2002) *Technology Appraisal Guidance No. 38: Nicotine Replacement Therapy (NRT) and Bupropion for Smoking Cessation*. London: National Institute for Clinical Excellence.

National Society for the Prevention of Cruelty to Children (1997a) Drunk in charge: substance abuse. *Community Care*, 11–17 September, 35.

—— (1997b) *NSPCC Calls for New Year's Resolution on Drinking*. Press release, 30 December 1998.

Nunes, E., Weissman, M., Goldstein, R., et al (1998) Psychopathology in children of parents with opiate dependence and/or major depression. *Journal of the American Academy of Child and Adolescent Psychiatry*, **37**, 1142–1151.

Nurco, D., Blatchley, R., Hanlon, T., et al (1999) Early deviance and related risk factors in the children of narcotic addicts. *American Journal of Drug and Alcohol Abuse*, **25**, 25–45.

O'Connor, M. J. & Kasari, C. (2000) Prenatal alcohol exposure and depressive features in children. *Alcohol Clinical and Experimental Research*, **23**, 1070–1076.

Rantakallio, P., Laara, E. & Koiranen, M. (1995) A 28 year follow up of mortality among women who smoked during pregnancy. *British Medical Journal*, **311**, 477–480.

Reich, W., Earls, F., Frankel, O., et al (1993) Psychopathology in children of alcoholics. *Journal of the American Academy of Child and Adolescent Psychiatry*, **32**, 995–1002.

Rickford, F. (1996) Bad habit. *Community Care*, 1–14 February, 16–17.

Scher, M., Richardson, G. A., Coble, P., et al (1988) The effects of prenatal alcohol and marijuana exposure: disturbances in neonatal sleep cycling and arousal. *Pediatric Research*, **24**, 101–105.

Schindler, S. D., Eder, H. & Ortner, R. (2003) Neonatal outcome following buprenorphine maintenance during conception and throughout pregnancy. *Addiction*, **98**, 103–110.

Scholl, T., Hediger, M. & Belsky, D. (1994) Prenatal care and maternal health during adolescent pregnancy: a review and meta analysis. *Journal of Adolescent Health*, **15**, 444–456.

Schuckit, M. A. (2000) Biological phenotypes associated with individuals at high risk for developing alcohol related disorders: Part II. *Addiction Biology*, **5**, 23–36.

—— & Smith, T. L. (2001) The clinical course of alcohol dependence associated with a low level of response to alcohol. *Addiction*, **96**, 903–910.

Scottish Executive (2001) *Policy and Practice Guidelines for Working with Children and Families Affected by Problem Drug Use*. Edinburgh: The Stationery Office.

Searles, I. & Windle, N. (1990) Introduction and overview: salient issues in the children of alcoholics literature. In *Children of Alcoholics: Critical Perspectives* (eds N. Windle & I. Searles), pp. 1–8. New York: Guildford.

Sher, K. (1997) Psychological characteristics of children of alcoholics. *Alcohol Health and Research World*, **21**, 247–254.

Steinhausen, H-C. (1995) Children of alcoholic parents: a review. *European Child and Adolescent Psychiatry*, **4**, 1143–1152.

Streissguth, A. P., Barr, H. M., Sampson, P. D., et al (1994a) Prenatal alcohol and offspring development: the first fourteen years. *Drug and Alcohol Dependence*, **36**, 89–99.

——, Sampson, H., Olson, H. C., et al (1994b) Maternal drinking during pregnancy: attention and short term memory in 14 year old offspring – a longitudinal prospective study. *Alcoholism: Clinical and Experimental Research*, **18**, 202–218.

Svikis, D. S., Golden, A. S., Huggins, G. R., et al (1997) Cost effectiveness of treatment for drug abusing pregnant women. *Drug and Alcohol Dependence*, **45**, 105–113.

Tronick, E. & Beeghly, M. (1999) Prenatal cocaine exposure, child development, and the compromising effects of cumulative risk. *Clinics in Perinatology*, **26**, 151–171.

Velleman, R. & Orford, J. (1999) *Risk and Resilience: Adults Who Were Children of Problem Drinkers*. Amsterdam: Harwood Academic Press.

Von Knorring, A-L. (1991) Annotation. Children of alcoholics. *Journal of Child Psychology and Psychiatry*, **32**, 411–421.

Weinberg, N. (1997) Cognitive and behavioural deficits associated with parental alcohol use. *Journal of the American Academy of Child and Adolescent Psychiatry*, **36**, 1177–1186.

West, M. O. & Prinz, R. (1987) Parental alcoholism and childhood psychopathology. *Psychological Bulletin*, **102**, 204–218.

Wilens, T., Biederman, J., Kiely, K., *et al* (1995) Pilot study of behavioural and emotional disturbances in the high-risk children of parents with opioid dependence. *Journal of the American Academy of Child and Adolescent Psychiatry*, **34**, 779–785.

Wisborg, K., Henriksen, T. B., Jespersen, L. B., *et al* (2000) Nicotine patches for pregnant smokers: a randomised controlled study. *Journal of Obstetrics and Gynaecology*, **96**, 967–971.

Woodby, L. L., Windsor, R. A., Snyder, S., *et al* (1999) Predictors of cessation during pregnancy. *Addiction*, **94**, 283–292.

Working Party of the Royal College of Psychiatrists and the Royal College of Physicians (2000) *Drugs, Dilemmas and Choices*. London: Gaskell.

Young, N. (1997) Effects of alcohol and other drugs on children. *Journal of Psychoactive Drugs*, **29**, 23–42.

CHAPTER 8

Health issues

Ilana B. Crome, Daphne Rumball and Mervyn London

Key points

- Health professionals must have a sound knowledge of the adverse health consequences of substance misuse in order to detect, treat and refer young people for adequate health care. The ability to carry out an assessment in an empathic non-judgemental manner is essential.
- The long-term accumulative effects of substance misuse may damage a young person's health. However, it is the acute impact, such as occurs during intoxication or overdose, that frequently causes more widespread damage. This is often complicated by the setting within which this occurs and the young person's lack of judgement and experience.
- Risks to health are often complicated by associated behaviour, such as sexual activity and dependency needs.
- Prevention and treatment may be influenced by issues of consent. Advice must be accurate and appropriate for young people.
- Young people often consume a mixture of alcohol and drugs. An overdose may not be accidental and the assessment should always cover suicidal intent and deliberate self-harm.
- Young people may take substances by swallowing, smoking, inhaling or injecting into a vein or under the skin. They may have minimal knowledge of the risks involved or of the safer practices used by older substance misusers.
- Despite the relatively shorter duration of use, young people are at risk of the same health complications as adults, particularly in the presence of dependent or excessive substance misuse. Adequate assessment and treatment are therefore essential.

Introduction

Health professionals have a key role in the identification and treatment of the physical and psychological problems related to substance misuse. It is not only the risk of considerable acute and chronic morbidity and mortality but also their unpredictability that make the health consequences significant.

However, health professionals also have a role in the prevention of health problems, in the maintenance of good health, and in minimising the health risks associated with substance misuse. They should, for example, give information about diet, hygiene and dental care. Furthermore, they may act as advocates or facilitate access to treatment services for physical disorder by vulnerable substance misusers, who may feel stigmatised and marginalised by the medical profession. Young people are at particular risk and are therefore in need of much support. Their pattern of use (e.g. binge drinking) may lead to intoxication, injury, accidents and even death (Bonomo *et al*, 2001; *Lancet*, 2001). They may be at risk through inexperience, for example with injecting techniques or cleaning equipment. They may be unaware of the likely acute and chronic physical health consequences of substance misuse, or of the need for safer sexual practices.

Many young substance users are ambivalent about their well-being. Health advice which focuses on negative or long-term outcomes is therefore less likely to be effective than that which focuses on their strengths and positive health outcomes.

Young people use substances for a host of social reasons. However, they may also use substances for the alleviation of emotional or physical pain, to counteract the effects or side-effects of prescribed or over-the-counter medication, and for weight reduction.

Socially deprived youngsters may, in addition, lack a structured and supportive social network, which might otherwise enable access to appropriate use of health services. Health professionals in touch with teenagers require an awareness of the relationship between substance misuse and physical problems, and an empathic, non-judgemental attitude, as well as the knowledge and skills to detect, treat and refer. These skills include immunisation, screening and prenatal care.

The harm that substances inflict is related to the physiological or pharmacological impact of one substance alone or in combination with other substances. It is also related to the quantity, 'quality' (adulterants, purity), route of administration, and duration of use, including severity of dependence. The 'set' (i.e. individual susceptibility to) and expectation of drug effects influences the young misuser, as does the 'setting' (i.e. the environment in which the drugs are taken) (Zinberg, 1984).

In this chapter the focus is on potentially life-threatening physical problems resulting from intoxication and withdrawal, as well as the longer-term health effects of substance misuse, which usually (although not always) accrue after heavy use of long duration. Since emergency medical services may be required and practitioners need to be aware of the presentations and consequences, the discussion centres on common clinical presentations, such as intoxication, withdrawal, smoking, injecting, overdose and bingeing. The influence of settings is explored. Comprehensive descriptions of physical health problems can be found in reviews (Saunders, 1991; Edwards & Peters, 1994; Royal College of Physicians, 2000; Ashton, 2001; Ghodse, 2002; Gowing *et al*, 2002; Edwards *et al*, 2003).

The mortality of excessive drinkers is at least twice that of the general population, and that of drug users up to 22 times higher. Substances affect every organ in the body: the central nervous, gastrointestinal, cardiovascular, respiratory, musculoskeletal and endocrine systems. Some problems (e.g. intoxication, withdrawal syndromes, deliberate overdose, injecting accidents, hypothermia, hyperthermia, dehydration and choking or suffocating) may require urgent medical attention.

Intoxication

Acute alcohol poisoning is greatly under-recognised as a risk and yet is the most common cause of substance-related death in young people. Acute intoxication with alcohol produces disinhibition, which, coupled with lack of judgement and coordination, makes users prone to accidents. With increasing quantities slurred speech, ataxia, blurred vision, decreased consciousness and even coma and death may result through choking, accident, hypoglycaemia or cerebral oedema.

Intoxication may, through a direct effect on behaviour, give rise to accidents, burns, falls, injuries and drowning. Young people who are very intoxicated will be cognitively impaired and will not be able to judge situations as dangerous; therefore they may wander into a busy road or fall off a building. Head injuries are common, and can affect how people tolerate and react to psychiatric medications. Head injuries also increase the risk of epileptic seizures, so caution needs to be taken when prescribing drugs that lower seizure threshold. People can lapse into deep sleep and choke on vomit. Hypothermia is a big risk for homeless drinkers, as alcohol reduces core body temperature.

Intoxication with opiates or alcohol causes diminished pain perception and therefore users can suffer serious injury without being aware of this (e.g. falling asleep next to a radiator after using heroin and receiving severe burns). Fire accidents may occur as a result of falling asleep after use of sedative drugs and leaving a cigarette burning or food cooking.

The link between violence and substance use is complex, but may partly be due to disinhibition. Young people, in particular, are prone to become aggressive if they feel frightened and trapped and if they misinterpret situations as hostile, for example when they are intoxicated or experiencing the after-effects of drugs. Alcohol and stimulant intoxication are particularly likely to increase aggression by disinhibition and increased irritability. Craving for substances and the physiological effects of withdrawal are also likely to increase agitation. Comorbid psychiatric illness can exacerbate substance-induced fear and paranoia.

Frightening or disturbing hallucinations and delusions can accompany the relapse of a mental illness and may occur in some withdrawal states. Acute intoxication may also mimic psychotic illness. Mental illnesses, including schizophrenia in the prodromal phase, may aggravate symptoms. Amphetamine, cocaine and cannabis may produce a range of psychotic symptoms.

The depressant effects of opiates on reflexes such as coughing and breathing can cause respiratory problems, including pneumonia. Fatal overdose is most common when a combination of drugs is used (e.g. alcohol and benzodiazepines). This may particularly be the case for novice users. Dangerous intoxication, especially in opiate users, may be precipitated by use after a period of abstinence and a consequently reduced tolerance. Thereafter the user experiences slow, shallow breathing, low blood pressure, altered consciousness, coma and death. Those who misuse benzodiazepines (which are often unrecognised as a problematic substance by users) may experience respiratory depression, dizziness, unsteadiness and cognitive impairment.

The health consequences should be noted of using easily obtainable substances for inducing intoxication, such as lighter fuel, petrol, glue and aerosols. Unsteadiness and incoordination typically result. Death may result from cardiac arrhythmias, or from accidents during intoxication. Fatalities as a result of the use of such substances for intoxication occur in about 75 young people each year in the UK.

Hypothermia may result from sleeping rough and being intoxicated with alcohol. Hyperthermia, notably from ecstasy use, may be accompanied by fits, circulatory problems, muscle damage, and renal and liver impairment. Indeed, there is a correlation between body temperature and the risk of mortality from ecstasy (Gowing *et al*, 2002).

Withdrawal

Specific syndromes arise as a result of alcohol and benzodiazepine withdrawal. Short-term alcohol withdrawal (i.e. 4–6 hours after the last drink) results in nausea, vomiting, sweating, malaise, insomnia and a coarse tremor. More severe symptoms, including illusions, convulsions, cardiac arrhythmias, hypertension and hyperthermia, occur after 12–36 hours. Although such syndromes in young people reflect unusually high levels of consumption, it is not uncommon for these health problems to emerge later in life after prolonged use. At its worst, the withdrawal syndrome features delirium tremens, which is characterised by tremor, extreme agitation, confusion, delusions and hallucinations. This may be mistaken for other confusional states or psychotic illness. Those suffering from such confusional states need psychiatric and medical care owing to risks of accidental harm, disturbed behaviour and also the risk of morbidity and mortality. People affected are typically disorientated as to where they are, the day and the date. They may act upon visual, tactile and auditory hallucinations. They may have short-term memory problems and be extremely distressed and frightened. Assessment should identify the cause of the delirium and treatment should focus on the underlying cause as well as the associated behavioural disorder.

In the unusual event of medical care not being directly available, the best short-term advice to a heavy drinker is to continue to drink alcohol at a minimum level and to cut down gradually, to prevent a withdrawal syndrome. For any young person requesting immediate help for alcohol withdrawal it is important to consider the high risk of suicide. Although delirium tremens is very uncommon in young people, it is potentially fatal (in adults, even if treated, it has a 15% mortality rate). Delirium tremens should be differentiated from organic damage through drinking causing a confused agitated state such as Wernicke's encephalopathy. It should be noted that convulsions may result owing to withdrawal or trauma, as well as cerebral and cerebellar atrophy.

Benzodiazepine dependence is associated with a withdrawal syndrome similar to that for alcohol, and carries a risk of fits.

Withdrawal from opiates, on the other hand, although very uncomfortable, is not usually life threatening. It leads to muscle aches and pains, goose-flesh, watering eyes and nose, sweating and diarrhoea. Rarely, prolonged diarrhoea and vomiting can cause death through dehydration and electrolyte loss, especially if associated with other physical illness. Young people may be more fearful of these withdrawal symptoms than older, more experienced opiate users. This anxiety may itself reinforce continued opiate use. Opiate withdrawal may be complicated by withdrawal from other substances, especially in custodial settings. Insomnia may persist for weeks, but other symptoms resolve in about a week, depending on the opiate used.

Withdrawal from stimulant drugs may lead to depression and inertia, and even suicidal ideas.

Smoking and inhalation

Smoking is used as a method for the consumption of nicotine, heroin, crack cocaine and cannabis, and volatile gases are used by inhalation (Hall & MacPhee, 2002). These methods of use may have an irritant effect on the respiratory system and exacerbate any underlying disorders, including asthma. Presentation with chronic cough is common.

Tobacco smoking is by far the most important cause of chronic bronchitis, and tests of lung function indicate that many young smokers have already developed narrowing of their small airways. In Western countries cancer of the lung is the most important of the cancers caused by tobacco. However, cigarette smoking can also cause cancers of the pancreas, bladder, oesophagus and cervix. It should also be noted that cigarettes cause more deaths from coronary artery disease and stroke than from cancer. Smoking decreases fertility. Young women who smoke during pregnancy increase the risk of stillbirth and neonatal death, and their children are subject to delay in physical and intellectual development. Furthermore, non-smokers are at risk of inhaling the smoke from those around them. Nicotine is the most significant gateway drug to other problematic substance use.

Evidence is accumulating with regard to those respiratory consequences of cannabis use that can be separated from nicotine use (Baldwin *et al*, 1997; Ashton, 2001; Hall, 2001). In addition, some substances, particularly opiates, have a direct suppressive effect on respiratory function and can cause death or chronic illness as a consequence, especially in combination with other depressant substances, such as alcohol and benzodiazepines. Chronic snorting of cocaine can lead to nose bleeds and to perforation of the nasal septum secondary to vasoconstriction.

Injecting

Injecting is mostly associated with the use of heroin, amphetamine or cocaine. However, most drugs (even alcohol) can be injected directly into the veins. Intravenous injecting carries a number of risks to health, and often the young user lacks the information and skills to inject in a manner that minimises those risks. A toxic dose is easily administered and takes effect immediately, so that instant death may be associated with injecting cocaine or crack as well as heroin.

Injecting carries risks of infection with the blood-borne viruses HIV, hepatitis B and hepatitis C. The risk occurs when injecting or preparing drugs using equipment contaminated with the blood or other body fluids of an infected person. Users are often unaware that 'sharing risks' relate to all paraphernalia, including spoons, water and filters, as well as needles and syringes. The hepatitis C virus is particularly infective and resistant to drying and cleaning. The risk is increased with the duration of injecting. Re-infection with other strains of the same virus or co-infection with other blood-borne viruses worsens prognosis (Department of Health, 2001a).

The risks of infection with a blood-borne virus are particularly high at the stage of initiation to injecting. There is also increased risk in the context of adolescent reckless behaviour and intoxication due to inexperience. Between 40% and 60% of individuals who have ever injected are positive for hepatitis C and 52% show exposure to the hepatitis B virus (Department of Health, 2001b). About 80% of those who contract hepatitis C will remain infected and have a long-term increased prevalence of cirrhosis, liver failure and cancer. Chronic infection with the hepatitis C virus also has multi-system effects, including loss of energy, depression, arthritis and vascular disorders. Five per cent of those who acquire hepatitis B, and 20% of those with a chronic infection, will develop cirrhosis or liver cancer. Between 152 000 and 228 000 drug users in the UK are currently infected with the hepatitis C virus, but there is a much larger pool of infected former users. However, certain types of hepatitis C infections have a good outcome if treated early. Detection and investigation have obvious benefits.

Septicaemia can result from bacterial infection through injecting and is life threatening. The symptoms include fever, loss of consciousness and a red rash. Accumulation of infected material in body tissues can cause localised infections in the central nervous system and within the heart. Particles of infected matter can also cause embolic tissue damage. Suspicion of septicaemia or its complications demands hospitalisation of the patient and the intravenous administration of antimicrobial agents.

There has been a recent spate of septicaemias with anaerobic organisms such as clostridium, which can cause catastrophic paralysis and death unless treated very promptly. Intravenous drug users are advised to seek urgent medical attention for abscesses and for sudden symptoms of blurred vision or weakness.

Fungal infections have been detected among injecting drug users. These are thought to be due to intravenous introduction of spores within contaminants such as lemon juice, which is used to increase the solubility of heroin. Severe fungal infection is prone to occur in the eye and results in loss of sight.

Repeated injecting is likely to damage the veins. Young women seem especially prone to this. Unskilled users commonly present with localised thrombophlebitis, abscesses and ulcers with a relatively short history of injecting. Injection into larger vessels in the groin (sometimes used to conceal evidence of injecting), calf or neck can lead to a deep-vein thrombosis. Urgent medical treatment must be sought to prevent further injury to the limb, and to prevent a cerebral or pulmonary embolism. A blockage of blood supply to a limb can also be caused by injection into an artery (e.g. of crushed tablets or irritant substances). This can lead to gangrene and loss of that limb or digit, or massive local tissue loss.

Young people are often introduced to injecting with minimal knowledge of the risks and poor access to safer equipment. They often allow other people to inject them and have little knowledge of the nature or quantity of the substance. The availability of needle exchange for under-18s involves complex issues of consent and appropriateness of advice. Young women appear to take greater risks with personal partners and many young men are introduced to injecting within the criminal justice system. Advice about avoidance of sharing and about safer techniques needs to be very specific and requires knowledge of common practices.

Overdose and self-harm

Accidental or deliberate overdose with sedatives, such as heroin, benzodiazepines and alcohol, may lead to collapse, loss of consciousness, coma and death; the use of stimulants, such as cocaine and amphetamines, may lead to a fast heart rate (tachycardia), irregular heart beats (arrhythmias) and the heart might stop beating (cardiac arrest). Mixing drugs to which the user is separately tolerant can lead to accidental overdose. This is usually as a result of mixing sedative drugs, when users would typically lapse into unconsciousness and coma. It is important for effective medical treatment that the paramedics or accident and emergency staff know what drugs have been consumed. Any drugs and bottles, pills and powders found near the collapsed person will help identify what has been used and should therefore be transported with them.

Overdose with illicit substances is commonly assumed to be accidental. However, this is often not the case and an association with suicidal ideas is common (Neale, 2000). Young people who overdose in any circumstances should receive a careful assessment of their mental state.

Suicidal ideas and impulses can be a result of craving for drugs, disinhibition, or exacerbation of distress as a result of intoxication. The National Confidential Enquiry into Suicide and Homicide emphasised that substance misuse is a very strong predictor of completed suicide (Appleby *et al*, 1997).

Deliberate self-harm is a term used to refer to behaviour that results in physical harm to the self as a way of coping with distressing feelings, but which does not result in death; in many cases deliberate self-harm is not even an attempt to end life. It may occur in response to a crisis, stress or a deterioration in mental state. Alternatively, such behaviours may arise in severe and enduring mental illness as a serious attempt to end one's life, or may occur while intoxicated with drugs. It is also argued that drug use, especially long-term alcohol use and injecting behaviour, constitutes a form of deliberate self-harm in itself. Common behaviours include lacerating body parts with sharp objects, inserting objects into the body, pulling hair out or hitting oneself. Reckless high-risk behaviour may also occur, for example walking out in front of fast traffic or jumping off a tall building. Some people report that their use of drugs reduces the desire to self-harm. In a situation of enforced abstinence (custody, psychiatric admission), and its ensuing distress, such behaviour is liable to return. It is vital to consider and advise about the possibility of accidental overdose due to reduced tolerance following discharge from hospital, prison or youth custody.

Those with a history of deliberate self-harm are more likely to complete suicide. Serious self-harm in a state of extreme agitation becomes a psychiatric emergency, and staff have a duty of care to prevent harm and reduce distress. A common assumption is that deliberate self-harm is a way of seeking attention and manipulation. However, such attributions may be applied to justify decisions (e.g. disengagement from a client) and this should be resisted. Deliberate self-harm may be used as a coping mechanism and thus to be told to stop can feel very frightening. This may lead to a build-up of tension and distress, leading to a more serious outcome such as completed suicide. Cutting and self-harm have common aetiological and risk factors with substance use.

Bingeing and chronic substance use

The safe limits on alcohol consumption have been estimated in studies of adult populations. Safe limits for younger people are probably much lower. Women are more susceptible to alcoholic liver disease. Even low levels of alcohol consumption increase the progression of liver damage in people with hepatitis C.

Harmful or dependent use of alcohol may directly affect the health of the young person or emerge in later life. Alcohol affects the central and peripheral nervous system. Alcohol-dependent people may be malnourished, as they get calories from alcohol alone. Thiamine deficiency may lead to Wernicke's encephalopathy or Korsakoff's syndrome. Wernicke's encephalopathy consists of ocular palsies, a confusional state and ataxia. This may develop into Korsakoff's syndrome, with short-term memory loss and disorientation in place and time, with confabulation and apathy. Some degree of reversibility is possible. Peripheral neuropathy, leading to numbness, incoordination and ataxia, is very common in chronic alcohol misusers. Alcoholic blackouts or transient episodes of loss of memory are particularly associated with binge and chronic drinking. Cerebellar atrophy causes difficulty in gait.

Alcohol use can lead to gastritis, ulcers and oesophageal varices. This may impede digestion, and cause nausea and vomiting and pain. Nutritional deficiency results. The liver may be affected initially by fatty change, later by alcoholic hepatitis and, finally, by cirrhosis. Sometimes this progresses to cancer. It should be noted that consumption levels and poor diet affect outcome. Alcohol also causes pancreatitis, which in turn may lead to diabetes and chronic abdominal pain. Alcohol use is associated with cancers of the digestive tract.

Excessive drinking increases the risk of cardiac problems, such as hypertension, stroke (haemorrhagic and thrombotic), cardiac arrhythmias and cardiomyopathy. Red blood cells enlarge and, owing to liver disease, production of clotting factor is impaired. Chronic bleeding from the stomach or gut may lead to iron-deficiency anaemia. If liver biopsy is considered, this may be contraindicated until alcohol use is reduced.

The reproductive system is affected directly by alcohol use, due to the effects of liver disease on hormonal metabolism. Fertility is reduced and breast enlargement is a consequence. Facial flushing occurs after alcohol use. There is a distinctive form of psoriasis related to alcohol use, and there are chronic effects (spider naevi, telangiectasia, palmar erythema) related to liver damage. Alcohol may also exacerbate acne.

Long periods of stimulant use lead to malnutrition, vitamin deficiencies, weight loss, and, in the case of ecstasy, dental problems, liver damage and kidney damage. In addition stroke, hypertension, cardiac dysrhythmias, convulsions and chest pain may develop. Chronic opiate use causes constipation in addition to lack of appetite, weight loss and nutritional deficiencies. Hypothermia, as a result of sleeping rough and being intoxicated with alcohol, and hyperthermia, after taking ecstasy, may lead to death. Dehydration, choking and suffocating while heavily sedated, or after sniffing aerosols, can be fatal.

Prolonged misuse of drugs such as ecstasy, stimulants, hallucinogens or alcohol may cause a range of unpredictable psychiatric symptoms, including mood swings, agitation, irritability and derealisation. Recovery may be gradual despite abrupt cessation of drug use. Ecstasy may result in a spectrum of neurotoxic effects, from short-term memory impairment to irreversible brain damage. This does not appear to be related to an extensive history of use.

Sexual behaviour and substance use

The associations between substance use and sexual exploitation, sexual abuse and prostitution have been outlined in Chapter 5, as have the effects of substance use in pregnancy (Chapter 7). The links between substance use and sexual behaviour are complex. Higher levels of injection sharing occur with intimate partners and it is more difficult to cease use if the partner is also using substances.

Access to primary prevention, screening and treatment is reduced in substance-using populations, even though they are at increased risk of infections and complications such as pelvic inflammatory disease and cervical cancer. Risks of acquiring HIV and hepatitis B are increased by co-infection with other sexually transmitted infections.

Sexual orientation is often an evolving issue during adolescence. Unresolved issues and feelings of stigma are known to be associated with substance use, particularly alcohol, and with higher risk of suicide.

Fertility is reduced by multiple factors, including the direct effects of opiates, nicotine and alcohol, poor diet and drug-related weight loss. However, women may occasionally ovulate despite amenorrhoea, and fertility can rapidly improve during treatment. Timely advice and treatment are therefore required. It is often assumed that contraceptive advice is appropriate when in fact the young woman is ambivalent or desiring pregnancy. Open discussion may not occur if censure is anticipated. Skill in this area is vital, as pregnancy or the desire to be pregnant may be a strong motivating factor for change, and unplanned or concealed pregnancy is likely to be problematic.

Diet and eating

Eating disorders are linked to the misuse of a wide range of substances, including over-the-counter medicines, particularly laxatives and opiates. Weight loss is easily explained by stimulant or other substance use. The underlying eating disorder and any associated psychiatric illness can therefore be easily missed. Many young people who become involved in substance use have little experience of good personal care and little opportunity to ensure that they have an adequate diet.

Taking account of the setting

The vulnerability of young people in both the child care and the custodial system illustrates the influence of the setting on the detection and treatment of health problems, especially when the effects of substance withdrawal compound anxiety, irritability and depression. The ending of statutory responsibility as young people emerge from the child care system entails a loss of surrogate parental figures. Detection of dependency is impaired by assumed or real adverse consequences which inhibit help seeking. Young prisoners are at high risk of substance-related withdrawal complications, unsafe substance use, exploitation and suicide. The rate of new infections with blood-borne viruses is significantly higher in the prison population, and the rate of immunisation against hepatitis B is inadequate. For those substance users at risk of being remanded in custody, immunisation is a particularly important intervention. The risk of overdose is increased in the period following release, as it is following discharge from treatment services.

Conclusion

The interaction between substance use and health is complex. The effects may be very rapid or insidious, by a direct pharmacological or physiological action, or indirect, owing to associated behaviours. Practitioners working with young substance misusers need to be aware of the relationship of substance misuse to a history of physical or psychological problems such as trauma, coma, confusion, delirium, memory problems, fever, agitation, convulsions, tremor, paranoia and hallucinations. This sensitivity or high index of suspicion may connect previous difficulties to a current acute presentation for which life-saving measures are required. For these reasons, it is obligatory to establish whether recent substance use, including the types, quantities, route and the time course of use, has a bearing on overt and covert physical and psychological symptoms. Even where the incidence of serious adverse effects is low, it is the unpredictability of those events that makes the health consequences significant.

References

Appleby, L., Shaw, J., Amos, T., *et al* (1997) *Safer Services: Report of the National Confidential Inquiry into Suicide and Homicide by People with Mental Illness.* London: The Stationery Office.

Ashton, H. (2001) Pharmacology and effects of cannabis: a brief review. *British Journal of Psychiatry*, **178**, 101–106.

Baldwin, G. C., Tashkin, D. P., Buckley, D. M., *et al* (1997) Habitual smoking of marijuana and cocaine impairs alveolar macrophage function and cytokine production. *Journal of Respiratory Critical Care Medicine*, **156**, 1606–1613.

Bonomo, Y., Coffey, C., Wolfe, R., *et al* (2001) Adverse outcomes of alcohol use in adolescents. *Addiction*, **96**, 1485–1496.

Department of Health (2001a) *Hepatitis C – Guidance for Those Working with Drug Users.* London: Department of Health.

—— (2001b) *Prevalence of HIV and Hepatitis Infections in the United Kingdom.* London: Department of Health.

Edwards, G. & Peters, T. J. (eds) (1994) Alcohol and alcohol problems. *British Medical Bulletin*, **50**.

——, Marshall, E. J. & Cook, C. C. H. (2003) *The Treatment of Drinking Problems: A Guide for the Helping Professions* (4th edn). Cambridge: Cambridge University Press.

Ghodse, A. H. (2002) *Drugs and Addictive Behaviour: A Guide to Treatment* (3rd edn). Cambridge: Cambridge University Press.

Gowing, L. R., Henry-Edwards, S. M., Irvine, R. J., *et al* (2002) The health effects of ecstasy. *Drug and Alcohol Review*, **21**, 53–63.

Hall, W. (2001) Reducing the harms caused by cannabis use: the policy debate in Australia. *Drug and Alcohol Dependence*, **62**, 163–174.

—— & MacPhee, D. (2002) Cannabis and cancer. *Addiction*, **97**, 243–247.

Lancet (2001) Editorial. Children and EtoH – the dangers need spelling out. *Lancet*, **358**, 343.

Neale, J. (2000) Suicidal intent in non-fatal illicit drug overdose. *Addiction*, **95**, 85–93.

Royal College of Physicians (2000) *Nicotine Addiction in Britain*. London: Royal College of Physicians.

Saunders, J. (1991) The physical complications of alcohol abuse. In *The International Handbook of Addiction Behaviour* (ed. I. B. Glass), pp. 135–140. London: Routledge.

Zinberg, N. (1984) *Drug Set and Setting: The Basis for Controlled Intoxicant Use*. New Haven: Yale University Press.

CHAPTER 9

Young people and smoking

Kate Woodhouse

Key points

- Tobacco use is the leading behavioural cause of poor health, early death and health inequality in the UK.
- The process of becoming a smoker is complex, but dependence appears to develop rapidly. By the mid-teens nearly one in four young people are smoking at least weekly, most of these every day, with girls apparently at greater risk.
- Nicotine has complex effects on mental function. Quitting often disrupts mood and concentration, and most young people believe that smoking itself controls anxiety, and this is a further barrier to cessation.
- Smoking is strongly linked with other substance use and with poor mental health, each perhaps reinforcing the other, yet treatment services rarely address tobacco use. In particular, smoking as a youth may be a risk factor for poor mental health in adult life.
- At the population level, 'quit smoking' campaigns are unlikely to have a major impact, and isolated prevention programmes seldom do more than delay the onset of regular smoking.
- As with other substance use, integrated population strategies, such as the US state-wide programmes, appear to be most effective.
- Given growing recognition of the links between deprivation, smoking, poor mental health and the use of substances other than tobacco, workers in these fields have valuable insights to share, from the clinical to the political level.

Introduction

In many ways, youth smoking occupies an anomalous position. Tobacco use is not illegal, and not directly linked to other major criminality; neither does it cause intoxication or obvious acute harm. Youth smoking therefore generates less public anxiety and clinical interest than alcohol or other substance use. Yet tobacco use is the leading behavioural cause of death – it roughly doubles risk throughout adult life – and also plays a major role in creating health inequality (Peto *et al*, 1994). The great majority of users start in their teens, including around 3000 a week in Britain alone, setting up lasting patterns of individual and community risk (Royal College of Physicians, 1992).

Smoking has been a major focus of health promotion initiatives. This has led to a broad range of population and individual interventions for both adults and young people; the US state-wide programmes are integrated population strategies perhaps unmatched in other areas of public health.

This chapter presents a broad summary of current perspectives, including the impact of early smoking, the extent of smoking among the young, potential influences on behaviour, and options for prevention. There are, of course, complex links between smoking and the use of other substances, but a review has not been attempted here.

The impact of youth smoking

Although acute harm is seldom apparent, youth smoking affects both current well-being and later disease risk. Perhaps most crucially, those who start early also tend to smoke heavily as adults and are least likely to stop (Elders *et al*, 1994).

Smoking accelerates the processes that manifest as disease in adult life. For example, young smokers already show abnormal blood fat profiles and more pronounced arterial damage. Cancer risk is disproportionately increased by early smoking and lung development is impaired, particularly for girls, which increases the later risk of chronic obstructive pulmonary disease (US Department of Health and Human Services, 2001). Since smoking is strongly associated with poor mental health, smoking-related conditions contribute substantially to excess mortality among adult psychiatric patients (Phelan *et al*, 2001).

Young smokers also have worse immediate health, both physically and mentally. Smoking at least doubles the risk of symptoms such as cough and wheeze, increases the risk of respiratory infections, and increases discomfort on exercise (Royal College of Physicians, 1992). Young smokers have more sick-days, and are more prone to stomach pain, headache and tiredness, although such disorders may also reflect emotional or family problems. Young women who smoke tend to suffer worse and longer-lasting menstrual pain (US Department of Health and Human Services, 2001). The mental health aspects of smoking are discussed further below.

Particularly for less-affluent youngsters, the cost of tobacco may limit other choices that might benefit well-being. However, for the young smokers themselves these drawbacks may seem minor in relation to the perceived benefits – in controlling mood, making friends and exploring new roles. Young people who feel distressed, isolated or confused may therefore find smoking particularly attractive.

Prevalence of youth smoking

As with other substance use, smoking may at first be highly context dependent, and the process of acquisition is complex. However, population prevalence gives a useful measure of public health.

By the age of 11 years, around a third of children in England have tried a cigarette, but only one in 100 smokes every week. Experimentation increases rapidly around 11–13 years, which suggests that sales laws are ineffective (in the UK it is illegal to sell tobacco to anyone under the age of 16 years) and by age 15 around two-thirds have tried (Office for National Statistics, 2000). 'Regular' smoking, meaning at least weekly, generally appears around the age of 12–15 years, with an overall prevalence of around one in eight by age 14 and almost one in four by age 15. Thus nearly half of those who experiment become regular users. By age 15 nearly all 'weekly' smokers are in fact smoking every day, a behaviour that tends to be stable. Standard data on weekly smoking may therefore obscure the real increase in tobacco dependence.

In total, around a tenth of those aged 11–16 years smoke regularly, a figure broadly unchanged over the past 20 years, despite a steady downtrend among adults. Prevalence appeared to fall from a peak in the mid-1990s, but data for 2001 showed that the trend was not consistent, as 10% were again recorded as being regular smokers (Office for National Statistics, 2002).

In many developed countries girls are now more likely to smoke than boys, and the consistency of this difference suggests it arises by more than chance (see below). The data for 2001 show that in England a third more girls than boys smoke regularly at age 11–16. There is a lack of population data on smoking among young people with mental health problems, although a recent review describes high adult rates, especially among those living in institutions (McNeill, 2001).

The following sections look at individual and policy aspects of youth smoking, and the implications for prevention.

Individual smoking behaviour

Nicotine dependence obviously plays a role in smoking, but this is in turn shaped by complex social and cultural influences. Initiation appears to depend largely on immediate needs and feelings (Brynin, 1999). A wide range of factors then influence the development of regular smoking or impede attempts to quit, and these are likely to act more strongly on young people with mental health or substance use problems.

Studies mainly from northern Europe and the United States describe the following associations between smoking and individual circumstances. Yet although such findings can inform individual practice, they explain little of the variance in the uptake of smoking. The complexity of influences also suggests that isolated interventions are unlikely to create effective population strategies (Stead *et al*, 1996).

The development of dependence

Nicotine dependence is itself classified as a psychiatric disorder, along with other forms of substance use. A review by the Royal College of Physicians (2000) rated nicotine as 'highly addictive, to a degree similar or in some respects exceeding addiction to "hard" drugs such as heroin or cocaine'.

Dependence is apparent among occasional and weekly smokers, although the relative importance of nicotine exposure and initial sensitivity is unclear. Tolerance can begin to develop after a first dose, and dependence may also develop rapidly; for example, a US survey found that within weeks a quarter of young monthly smokers showed signs of dependence, and a few did so within days (DiFranza *et al*, 2000). In Britain a third of young 'weekly' smokers reach for a cigarette within half an hour of waking (which is a measure of dependence among adults) and only a minority would find it 'very easy' not to smoke for a day (Barton, 1998). Young people who smoke every day take as much nicotine from each cigarette as adults, and suffer similar withdrawal symptoms. US research suggests an increasing degree of dependence among the young, despite falling prevalence there. This also applies to British adults, as smoking becomes concentrated among those living with deprivation and poor psychological health (Hughes, 2001).

The development of dependence is subject to complex influences, including biological factors, although the exact mechanisms are poorly understood (Clayton *et al*, 2000). Both behavioural and biological studies suggest that genetic traits play a role in the initiation and maintenance of smoking. Prenatal exposure strongly predicts later experimentation, independent of later maternal smoking (Cornelius *et al*, 2000). Young people also vary in initial physiological response; for example, girls suffer more discomfort at first, but persist, and may become more dependent given similar intake (Goddard, 1990).

The psychology of smoking

Young smokers greatly overestimate peer smoking, and although most acknowledge the health risk, they tend to see more benefits to smoking than do non-smokers. This particularly applies to the belief that smoking controls stress, which appears to be a major barrier to cessation. For example, nearly all teenage smokers in Britain feel smoking can help you keep calm, compared with a small minority of non-smokers (Barton, 1998). Some studies show that girls have more positive beliefs about smoking, particularly in relation to control of weight and mood. Young smokers generally have poorer emotional health (see below). However, some research has found that girls who smoke tend to be more confident than their peers.

The social context

The development of smoking behaviour may be seen in relation to four broad circles of influence – the family, peers, school and the wider community – with times of transition perhaps increasing risk.

Children's smoking is strongly affected by family culture. Smoking by any sibling quadruples the risk of starting, and smoking by both parents increases the risk around threefold (Office for National Statistics, 1997). On the other hand, parental disapproval or quitting reduces this risk. Peer influence gains importance from around the early teens, and transition to a new school can be a time of vulnerability. Girls tend to make a sharper transition to a smaller peer group, and are more influenced by best friends' behaviour (Goddard, 1990).

Smoking is also linked to poor educational achievement, and early school leaving strongly predicts adult tobacco use (Graham & Der, 1999). Young smokers tend to feel alienated from school, and have low expectations of success, perhaps reflecting the mood of hopelessness noted in poor communities with a high prevalence of smoking. Qualitative evidence suggests that young people in deprived areas may feel under great pressure to follow community norms, and research on adult smokers suggests a 'community risk factor', in addition to individual risk. While deprived teenagers are somewhat more likely to take up smoking, they are much less likely to quit before their early thirties, as more affluent groups tend to do. The transition to college or the workplace may also bring new risk, as a new culture is encountered, but these young adults are generally more motivated to stop than are the unemployed (Trevett, 1997).

Smoking and mental health

There are clear links between youth smoking and poor mental health, from mild mood disorders to severe mental illness. Smoking has been associated with low self-esteem, depression and anxiety, perhaps particularly among girls. Youth tobacco use is also linked with poor sleep, eating disorders, suicide attempts, hyperactivity and other problem behaviours (Patton, 1996; Tyas & Pederson, 1998). These issues are interrelated; for example, a survey of young women in Ottawa and London found strong links between smoking, very low self-esteem and eating disorders (Crisp *et al*, 1998). On the other hand, measures of good mental health, such as resilience and the ability to self-regulate and solve problems, appear to protect against the uptake of smoking (Braverman, 1999).

However, evidence on causation is complex (McNeill, 2001). Some prospective studies suggest that poor mental health (including depression, anxiety and hyperactivity) may predict smoking, even after adjustment for other factors, such as social class, but not vice versa. In some situations smoking may be seen as an attempt to self-medicate. This theory has been applied to adults with schizophrenia, for example to counter negative symptoms or the effects of medication, and to the link with depression and anxiety among teenagers (Patton, 1996). Other analyses suggest that smoking predicts poor mental health, but not the opposite. For example, recent studies suggest that teen smoking predicts anxiety disorders in the early twenties, and that current smoking is a strong predictor of developing severe depressive symptoms (Goodman & Capitman, 2000; Johnson *et al*, 2000). A further study suggests that youth smoking and depression mutually predict each other (Windle & Windle, 2001).

These problems may have common genetic, psychological and social antecedents. For example, the link between smoking and major depression has been explained as essentially genetic (Kendler *et al*, 1993). Other studies suggest the association may occur primarily via deprivation or other social factors (McGee *et al*, 1998). Such apparent inconsistencies may be due to differences between study groups.

Whatever the initial causation, smoking cessation is clearly linked to acute mood disturbance, both through withdrawal and perhaps through the effect of habit change and loss. Symptoms commonly include depression, anxiety, irritability and restlessness, with similar findings for adults and young people (Royal College of Physicians, 2000). Yet several studies have shown that, within weeks, adults who stop become calmer than continuing smokers (West & Hajek, 1997). On the other hand, depression may become severe, especially in those with a previous history, and apart from craving is the only withdrawal symptom that predicts relapse to smoking (Royal College of Physicians, 2000).

Other substance use

Smoking is clearly associated with the use of alcohol and other drugs. For example, regular drinking is strongly associated with smoking, especially among boys, and 'relief' smoking predicts later heavy drinking. Early smoking in particular appears to predict future substance use, and other health risk behaviours (Lewinsohn *et al*, 1999).

As with poor mental health, there are likely to be common mechanisms at work. Smokers and those with other substance use problems may share genetic traits. Tobacco use and other substance use appear to have common neural mechanisms, for example promoting dopamine release within the nucleus accumbens (Royal College of Physicians, 2000). Young people who are heavy users of tobacco and other substances show a similar pattern of poor educational achievement, deprivation and identification with a subgroup. Poor mental health, social difficulties, heavy smoking and other substance use may thus form a cluster of problems that tend to reinforce each other. This obviously presents a challenge for both individuals and organisations, with smoking usually taking lower priority.

Gender differences

There are as yet no clear explanations for the persistence of youth smoking, or for higher smoking rates among girls. Some explanations apply to both sexes, but perhaps affect girls more. For example, young people now mature earlier, within a youth culture that is tolerant or approving of some drugs. Social inequalities may have increased risk over recent decades, and there are signs of increasing psychosocial distress among the young.

Other influences may particularly affect girls. For example, young women show increasing concern with weight, looks and 'style', and often believe that smoking can control weight (US Department of Health and Human Services, 2001). Girls' dissatisfaction with their bodies rises sharply around the age of 11–15 years, perhaps triggering sudden loss of self-esteem, while boys become slightly happier with their physique (World Health Organization, 1999). Young women may also be more influenced by positive images of smoking in magazines. Yet several reviews conclude that the conflicts of adolescence also play a key role: individual or group member, active or passive, sexual being or good student? Young women may feel these tensions most sharply, and cigarettes perhaps seem to offer some resolution, being for young people 'both forbidden and normal, alternative and accessible' (Stead *et al*, 1996).

The policy context

Like adults, young people are strongly influenced by how tobacco is marketed. Response can be considered in terms of the classic issues of price, placing, product and promotions.

Access to tobacco – price and placing

At the population level, trends in teenage smoking follow price changes. Most but not all studies suggest the young are more price responsive than adults, although response may vary by gender, social group and level of involvement with tobacco (Chaloupka & Grossman, 1997). Despite sales laws, children and young people generally find it easy to buy tobacco; it is estimated that the tobacco industry made £35 million profit from illegal sales across the UK in 1997 (Action on Smoking and Health, 2002).

Creating demand – product and promotions

Nearly all customers for tobacco products are gained for life in their teens, and the tobacco industry has therefore been concerned to form early brand loyalty. That marketing and product characteristics are designed with 'starters' in mind is apparent from industry documents made public as a result of legal settlements (Action on Smoking and Health, 1998).

Young people are exposed to a wide range of marketing techniques. For example, magazines are a trusted source of health information, yet may include both promotions and positive editorial content. Hoardings and sports sponsorship place the brand name repeatedly before the young viewer, 'brand-stretching' links tobacco to other desirable goods, and around one in 12 British teenagers owns clothing with a tobacco logo (Barton, 1998). Finally, there is evidence that the tobacco industry has paid for 'product placement' in major films with youth appeal (Sargent et al, 2001).

Many types of study suggest a causal link between promotions and tobacco use. Most specifically, recent prospective studies show that those most exposed to promotions, for example by owning a promotional item, are two to three times more likely to progress to smoking than controls – an effect size that is comparable to the impact of parental smoking in multivariate analysis. This even applies to children who had insisted they would never smoke, which suggests that promotions do not simply trigger existing intent (Pierce et al, 1998).

The elements of prevention

Tackling smoking among the young must obviously go beyond traditional schools programmes: the complex influences on smoking suggest the need for coordinated strategies, including whole-population approaches (Stead et al, 1996). Such measures may be more effective before smoking is fully established, give a consistent social message, and also reduce adult smoking. Adult example is arguably a key factor, given the

121

problems in designing appropriate messages for this age group, and the poor results of many youth interventions (Hill, 1999).

Strategies can be seen in terms of the four levels of public health intervention:

- policy measures;
- the social context, modified via media and peer or community projects;
- personal education;
- service and community development, for example provision of cessation support.

Mental health and substance use workers arguably have a role at all these levels, although the potential is largely unexplored.

The 1998 government white paper *Smoking Kills* set out to encourage a comprehensive approach. However, a full youth programme has perhaps been lacking, and new policies have been suggested within the coronary prevention framework (National Heart Forum, 2002). On the global stage, the World Health Organization is developing a Framework Convention on Tobacco Control, which again proposes a comprehensive strategy to protect young people.

Policy measures

A wide range of policies affect youth demand or restrict access, although tobacco promotion and taxation appear to be the key issues. For example, a review concluded that higher prices are the single best method to reduce demand among both youths and adults (Jha & Chaloupka, 2000). In the UK, the annual government budgets give campaign groups an opportunity to press for an increase in real price, at the promised level of at least 5% a year, and gain media coverage, particularly of youth smoking.

Youth access is also restricted by legislation forbidding sales to minors and restricting access to vending machines, and various campaigns have sought to improve local compliance. Current evidence suggests that prosecutions and linked publicity are more effective than staff training (Stead & Lancaster, 2001). However, such interventions are unlikely to have a large effect, as implementation is difficult, and young people simply get cigarettes elsewhere. School or workplace policies also in a sense restrict access, and give some evidence of reduced consumption. Psychiatric units are, of course, workplaces and, despite staff concerns, smoking policies within such units have generally been found acceptable to service users (Health Development Agency, 2000).

In relation to tobacco promotions, a World Bank report estimated that European Union legislation then proposed would reduce average consumption by around 7% across member states (Jha & Chaloupka, 1999). A review of the effects of advertising bans in Norway, Finland, New Zealand and France suggests that young people benefit substantially from such controls (Joossens, 2000). At the time of writing, a Private Member's Bill to control promotions is making good progress within Parliament, but the European legislation is still under discussion.

The social context

Young people are, of course, affected by many social influences, including media coverage. This has prompted attempts to shape the social climate through the use of paid media. Media-only campaigns targeted at the young have generally had limited impact, the few successful trials using substantial exposure of carefully designed messages (Sowden & Arblaster, 2000*a*). This issue has received little research, although US campaigns show promising results (see 'Integrated campaigns', below). Teenagers may also be influenced by paid media aimed at adults, and unpaid media coverage has a crucial role in setting the adult agenda, and in influencing policy and funding decisions.

Community-based campaigns aim to change the social climate within a locality. However, a stringent review concluded that only around a third of those that met criteria were successful (Sowden & Arblaster, 2000*b*). However, again the US campaigns suggest that well-funded initiatives can have a substantial impact.

Personal education

Youth smoking has traditionally been approached via school-based educational projects. Some major reviews have concluded that the more successful projects focus on social influence and skills, use active learning, and include short-term risks and wider health topics. Initiatives should also start at a young age, include booster contacts and ideally form part of a community project (Stead *et al*, 1996; NHS Centre for Reviews and Dissemination, 1999). However, even the best-designed projects sometimes prove ineffective, and few interventions do more than delay regular smoking, perhaps for up to ten years. A review of randomised controlled trials of school-based interventions concluded there was little good evidence on interventions linked to community projects, or combined social influences and social skills approaches. Among the best studies of 'social influences', only half showed a positive effect (Thomas, 2002). Most projects also prove impractical for large-scale use outside the research context, and with few exceptions appear less effective for girls.

There is obviously a role for educational projects, as young people have a right to information, and delayed smoking reduces health risk and predicts early cessation. However, these should form only part of wider initiatives, both nationally and within the school. For example, work on smoking might more effectively be linked to school smoking policies and work on other health issues, including mental health, perhaps within 'health-promoting schools' schemes.

Smoking cessation services

Many young smokers may intend to stop, although individual motivation fluctuates. For example, a national survey found that half of British teenage smokers wanted to quit, and very few were definitely not interested (Barton, 1998). Actual attempts to stop are frequent – the same survey found that two-thirds of the girls and half the boys had tried.

Guidelines for the UK suggest that young smokers should be offered the same support as adults, and the World Health Organization has also called for better services for this group (Raw et al, 1998). Adult guidelines recommend that health workers offer brief advice using the '4A' model – to ask, advise smokers to stop, assist if appropriate, and arrange follow-up. This might include referral to the specialist adviser system, which is now developing youth initiatives in some areas of the UK.

However, although young people have a right to such support, there is not yet clear evidence on its effectiveness (Foulds, 2000; Moolchan et al, 2000). Recruitment and retention tend to be difficult, as young people's motivation fluctuates, and the population impact is likely to be modest. British studies suggest that brief advice from a general practitioner may be acceptable to young people, although the role of other workers is largely untested, and helpline support is popular. Some organisations have run support groups for young smokers, and the charity QUIT is now piloting a national group scheme. The use of nicotine replacement therapy for young people is under review in two projects around Nottingham.

The role of mental health or substance use workers has hardly been explored, both groups obviously tending to have more immediate priorities. Yet clients themselves may be interested: for example, a review notes that in Britain around half the adult smokers with mental health problems would like to stop (McNeill, 2001). A limited body of work suggests that these smokers may benefit from cognitive–behavioural or group approaches. In general, smokers with mood problems may benefit from social support during cessation (US Department of Health and Human Services, 2001). The nicotine patch appears effective for adults diagnosed with schizophrenia and for women with a history of depression or anxiety. The antidepressants nortriptyline and bupropion also boost cessation rates among smokers generally, the latter apparently independent of its antidepressant effect. Few trials have looked specifically at the needs of young smokers with poor mental health, although brief motivational interviewing may offer some benefit (Colby *et al*, 1998).

At the very least, tobacco use should be mentioned in health resources and during individual discussion of needs, with referral to other services such as helplines or specialist advisers if appropriate. Smoking could also be given higher priority within mental health promotion for young people generally, as part of an integrated approach to health. For example, combined fitness and education sessions may both improve mood and reduce smoking rates (Collingwood *et al*, 2000).

Inequality

The role of inequality in shaping tobacco use is attracting growing interest, and initiatives such as the Scotland Inequalities project by Action on Smoking and Health are now developing work in poorer areas. For young people generally, the best long-term results may come from improved education and training opportunities (Graham & Der, 1999). However, wider social policy on employment, benefits, housing and child care will also ameliorate family poverty and linked risk. Some work suggests that even small improvements in individual circumstances can have a substantial impact on adult smoking rates, which should reduce risk among the young (Graham, 1998).

Integrated campaigns

Recent programmes within the United States have demonstrated the value of comprehensive and integrated approaches in reducing smoking across the age range. As a result of legal action against the tobacco industry, several states have gained access to unprecedented funds, and implemented multi-level programmes that feature policy, media, educational, community and cessation elements.

These campaigns have proved highly effective (Wakefield & Chaloupka, 2000). For example, the Californian programme nearly halved teenage smoking rates during 1995–99, down from 12.1% to 6.9%. Adult prevalence also halved, reducing low birth weight and cardiovascular events (Californian Department of Health Services, 2000). The programme saves around $3.60 for each dollar spent, solely in direct medical expenditure. Other regions of the world are investigating similar legal action; however, the initial costs will be beyond most countries, which can perhaps only aim for a similarly comprehensive approach.

Conclusion

The roots of youth smoking are complex, tightly interwoven and deeply embedded in adult culture. Isolated youth projects may therefore have limited long-term impact and may not be cost-effective, however politically attractive they are. Comprehensive population-wide measures are therefore essential, including:

- accessible cessation services;
- educational projects based on current research findings, and integrated within a broader health-promoting curriculum;
- work with media sources to challenge positive images of tobacco use;
- implementation of policy, especially to maintain real price and control tobacco promotions.

However, tobacco remains outside the scope of most substance use and mental health initiatives. Given the interlinked nature of these problems, it seems important that workers consider tobacco along with other substance use, support young smokers in aiming for cessation, and claim a larger role within policy development.

Acknowledgement

Grateful thanks to Dr Ann McNeill for comments on a draft of this chapter.

References

Action on Smoking and Health (1998) *Tobacco Explained: 3. Marketing to Children.* At http://www.ash.org.uk/html/conduct/html/tobexpld3.html
—— (2002) *Factsheet 3: Young People and Smoking.* At http://www.ash.org.uk/
Barton, J. (1998) *Young Teenagers and Smoking in 1997.* London: Office for National Statistics.
Braverman, M. T. (1999) Research on resilience and its implications for tobacco prevention. *Nicotine Tobacco Research,* 1 (suppl. 1), S67–S72.
Brynin, M. (1999) Smoking behaviour: predisposition or adaptation? *Journal of Adolescence,* 22, 635–646.
Californian Department of Health Services (2000) *California Tobacco Control Update.* Sacramento: Californian Department of Health Services.
Chaloupka, F. J. & Grossman, M. (1997) Price, tobacco control policies and smoking among young adults. *Journal of Health Economics,* 16, 359–373.
Clayton, R. R., Ries Merikangas, K. & Abrams, D. B. (eds) (2000) Tobacco, nicotine and youth. *Drug and Alcohol Dependence,* 59 (suppl 1).
Colby, S. M., Monti, P. M., Barnett, N. P., *et al* (1998) Brief motivational interviewing in a hospital setting for adolescent smoking. *Journal of Consulting and Clinical Psychology,* 66, 574–578.
Collingwood, T. R., Sunderhan, J., Reynolds, R., *et al* (2000) Physical training as a substance abuse prevention intervention for youth. *Journal of Drug Education,* 30, 435–451.
Cornelius, M. D., Leech, S. L., Goldschmidt, L., *et al* (2000) Prenatal tobacco exposure: is it a risk factor for early tobacco experimentation? *Nicotine Tobacco Research,* 2, 45–52.

Crisp, A. H., Halek, L., Sedgewick, P., et al (1998) Smoking and pursuit of thinness in schoolgirls in London and Ottawa. *Postgraduate Medical Journal*, **74**, 473–479.

DiFranza, J. R., Rigotti, N. A., McNeill, A. D., et al (2000) Initial symptoms of nicotine dependence in adolescents. *Tobacco Control*, **9**, 313–319.

Elders, M. J., Perry, C. I., Eriksen, M. P., et al (1994) The report of the Surgeon General: preventing tobacco use among young people. *American Journal of Public Health*, **84**, 543–547.

Foulds, J. (2000) *Smoking Cessation in Young People*. London: Health Development Agency.

Goddard, E. (1990) *Why Children Start Smoking*. London: HMSO.

Goodman, E. & Capitman, J. (2000) Depressive symptoms and cigarette smoking among teens. *Pediatrics*, **106**, 748–755.

Graham, H. (1998) Health at risk: poverty and national health strategies. In *Women and Health Services* (ed. L. Doyal), pp. 22–39. Milton Keynes: Open University Press.

— & Der, G. (1999) Influences on women's smoking status. *European Journal of Public Health*, **9**, 137–141.

Health Development Agency (2000) *Tobacco Control Policies Within Psychiatric and Long-stay Units – A Consultation Document*. London: Health Development Agency.

Hill, D. (1999) Why we should tackle adult smoking first. *Tobacco Control*, **8**, 333–335.

Hughes, J. R. (2001) Distinguishing nicotine dependence from smoking: why it matters to tobacco control and psychiatry. *Archives of General Psychiatry*, **58**, 817–818.

Jha, P. & Chaloupka, F. J. (1999) *Curbing the Epidemic: Governments and the Economics of Tobacco Control*. Washington, DC: World Bank.

— & — (2000) The economics of global tobacco control. *British Medical Journal*, **321**, 358–361.

Johnson, J. G., Cohen, P., Pine, D. S., et al (2000) Association between cigarette smoking and anxiety disorders during adolescence and early adulthood. *Journal of the American Medical Association*, **284**, 2348–2351.

Joossens, L. (2000) *The Effectiveness of Banning Advertising for Tobacco Products*. International Union Against Cancer – see http://www.ash.org.uk/html.advspo/html/experience.html.

Kendler, K. S., Neale, M. C., Maclean, C. J., et al (1993) Smoking and major depression – a causal analysis. *Archives of General Psychiatry*, **50**, 36–43.

Lewinsohn, P. M., Rohde, P. & Brown, R. A. (1999) Level of current and past cigarette smoking as predictors of future substance abuse disorders in young adulthood. *Addiction*, **94**, 913–921.

McGee, R., Williams, S. & Stanton, W. (1998) Is mental health in childhood a major predictor of smoking in adolescence? *Addiction*, **93**, 1869–1874.

McNeill, A. D. (2001) Smoking and mental health – a review of the literature. At http://www.ash.org.uk/html/policy/menlitrev.html.

Moolchan, E. T., Ernst, M. & Henningfield, J. E. (2000) A review of tobacco smoking in adolescents: treatment implications. *Journal of the American Academy of Child and Adolescent Psychiatry*, **39**, 682–693.

National Heart Forum (2002) *Towards a Generation Free From Coronary Heart Disease: Policy Action for Children's and Young People's Health and Well-being*. London: National Heart Forum. At www.heartforum.org.uk/childrenshealth.html.

NHS Centre for Reviews and Dissemination (1999) Can young people be prevented from taking up smoking? *Effective Health Care Bulletin*, **5**.

Office for National Statistics (1997) *Teenage Smoking Attitudes in 1996*. London: Office for National Statistics.

— (2000) *Drug Use, Smoking and Drinking Among Young Teenagers in 1999*. London: Stationery Office.

— (2002) *Living in Britain: Results from the 2001 General Household Survey*. London: Office for National Statistics.

Patton, G. C. (1996) Is smoking associated with depression and anxiety in teenagers? *American Journal of Public Health*, **86**, 225–230.

Peto, R., Lopez, A. D., Boreham, J., *et al* (1994) *Mortality from Smoking in Developed Countries 1950–2000*. Oxford: Oxford University Press.

Phelan, M., Stradius, L. & Morrison S. (2001) Physical health of people with severe mental illness. *British Medical Journal*, **322**, 443–444.

Pierce, J. P., Choi, U. S., Gilpin, E. A., *et al* (1998) Tobacco industry promotion of cigarettes and adolescent smoking. *Journal of the American Medical Association*, **279**, 511–515. Published erratum *JAMA*, **280**, 422.

Raw, M., McNeill, A. & West, R. (1998) Smoking cessation guidelines for health professionals, a guide to effective smoking cessation interventions for the health care system. *Thorax*, **53** (suppl. 5).

Royal College of Physicians (1992) *Smoking and the Young*. London: Royal College of Physicians.

— (2000) *Nicotine Addiction in Britain*. London: Royal College of Physicians.

Sargent, J. D., Tickle, J. J., Beach, M. L., *et al* (2001) Brand appearances in contemporary cinema films and contribution to global marketing of cigarettes. *Lancet*, **357**, 29–32.

Sowden, A. J. & Arblaster, L. (2000*a*) Mass media interventions for preventing smoking in young people (Cochrane Review). In *The Cochrane Library 4*, (2) CD001006. Oxford: Update Software.

— & — (2000*b*) Community interventions for preventing smoking in young people. (Cochrane Review). In *The Cochrane Library 4*, (2) CD001291. Oxford: Update Software.

Stead, L. F. & Lancaster, T. (2001) Interventions for preventing tobacco sales to minors (Cochrane Review). In *The Cochrane Library 4*, (1) CD001497. Oxford: Update Software.

Stead, M., Hastings, G. & Tudor-Smith, C. (1996) Preventing adolescent smoking: a review of the options. *Health Education Journal*, **55**, 31–54.

Thomas, R. (2002) School-based programmes for preventing smoking (Cochrane Review). In *The Cochrane Library, 1*. Oxford: Update Software.

Trevett, N. (1997) *Lighting Up: Smoking Among 16–24 Year Olds*. London: Health Education Authority.

Tyas, S. L. & Pederson, L. L. (1998) Psychosocial factors related to adolescent smoking: a critical review of the literature. *Tobacco Control*, **7**, 409–420.

US Department of Health and Human Services (2001) *Women and Smoking*. Bethesda, MD: US Department of Health and Human Services.

Wakefield, M. & Chaloupka, F. (2000) Effectiveness of comprehensive tobacco control programmes in reducing teenage smoking in the USA. *Tobacco Control*, **9**, 177–186.

West, R. & Hajek, P. (1997) What happens to anxiety levels on giving up smoking? *American Journal of Psychiatry*, **154**, 1589–1592.

Windle, M. & Windle, R. C. (2001) Depressive symptoms and cigarette smoking among middle adolescents: prospective associations and intrapersonal and inter-personal influences. *Journal of Consulting and Clinical Psychology*, **69**, 215–226.

World Health Organization (1999) *Gender and Health in Adolescence*. Copenhagen: World Health Organization.

CHAPTER 10

The process of assessment

Ilana B. Crome

Key points

- The objective of an assessment is to determine the use, misuse, harmful use or dependent use of the range of licit and illicit, prescribed and over-the-counter substances that the young person may be taking.
- Assessment should explore the effect of substance use on the young person's social, physical and psychological development as it relates to appropriate interventions, since almost always substance misuse is not the only problem.
- Adequate risk assessment includes child protection issues, suicide risk, extent of chaotic use and current accommodation.
- Consideration should be given to the hierarchy of needs: safety, accommodation, good care, education and therapeutic intervention.
- It is important to assess the maturity of the young person, as this affects consent to, or more importantly refusal of, treatment.
- The practitioner's core aspiration should be that the young person remains engaged, with the recognition that the assessment process is continuous.
- Further management should be based on the clinician's balanced interpretation of the systematic history, clinical condition and results of investigations.
- Communication of the assessment – to the young person, family and carers, and relevant professionals – is important.

Introduction

This chapter focuses on the process, the purpose and the practicalities of assessment. As well as providing an outline of the types of questions that must be asked to determine the treatment process, it also discusses the variety of settings, referral routes, and personal and wider social environments that may have an effect on assessment interviews. It starts from the premise that thorough history taking is fundamental to therapeutic objectives (Glass *et al*, 1991; Ghodse, 1995; Farrell *et al*, 1996; Edwards *et al*, 1997; Department of Health, 1999).

Thus it deals with information gathering from the patient and from other informants, and how this directs and clarifies decisions or judgements about treatment planning. It takes account of the way in which this assessment may be amplified by context, such as the maturity and vulnerability of the young person or the family situation. Discussion of how the mental state examination and further investigations may influence the assessment process then follows. Of course, in an emergency, the demands of the clinical situation may alter the course of events described.

Assessment aims to determine the use, misuse or harmful use of, or dependence on, the full range of prescribed, illicit and licit substances that the young person may be using. It should clarify the effect of this behaviour on the individual's social, psychological and physical development. In addition, it is necessary to distinguish, if possible, between symptoms, unresolved vulnerabilities and extrinsic factors that may precede, result in, or sustain substance use.

An adequate risk assessment, with particular consideration of child protection issues, but that also covers suicidal risk, episodes of deliberate self-harm, current accommodation and extent of chaotic use, is a vital component of the first interview, since emergency or urgent arrangements may have to be made. It is useful to bear in mind a hierarchy of needs: safety, accommodation, good care, education and then therapeutic intervention.

In this context, it is necessary to judge whether the young person is sufficiently mature to consent to or, more importantly, to refuse treatment. Clinical judgement of the motivation and expectations of the young person and family is also critical in determining how to proceed. Only after taking into account all facets will the clinician be in a position to initiate appropriate and effective therapies safely. This includes the coordination of subsequent meetings with the range of appropriate professionals in a manner that is least threatening to the young person. The practitioner's core aspiration should be to ensure that the young person remains engaged, with the recognition that the assessment process is a continuous one.

Referral routes

Young people may be referred to a range of different psychiatrists, including child and adolescent, forensic, liaison, learning disability and neuropsychiatrists and their teams, from a great diversity of sources. They may be referred from other medical practitioners (e.g. general practitioners, paediatricians and physicians); they may be directed by the social, educational or criminal justice services; often parents, family, friends and carers refer young people; and sometimes clients or patients even refer themselves.

Whatever the referral route, the consultation is likely to be a momentous event and to engender a degree of anxiety in the young person. The consultation should be undertaken in a pleasant, personal and private environment and the practitioner should adopt an accepting style; a balance should be struck between being serious and dull! A decision needs to be made with the young person as to whether significant others will participate in the interview, and at what point this might be desirable. The age and developmental maturity of the young person are important factors.

The setting of the first consultation

Emergency

The first consultation may be as a result of an emergency or crisis. Substance misusers in crisis are likely to contact a variety of health and social service agencies. Examples of such a crisis include an accident (e.g. road traffic accidents, falls, overdose or intoxication) or panic following a reaction to a substance. Presentation at services may also be part of drug-seeking behaviour.

Planned

The assessment is more likely to be planned if there has been a change in the young person's life that has precipitated a change in perception about substance use (e.g. problems at school, college or work, relationship difficulties, or legal problems).

Key considerations in assessment

Differentiation between use, misuse, harmful use and dependence

As has been discussed earlier in the book and in this chapter, the practitioner will need to be familiar with the differentiation between the use, misuse, harmful use and dependent use of substances:

Use	The term 'use' is applied to legal use, which is acceptable socially, medically approved and which is non-hazardous (i.e. without impairment of social, psychological or physical functioning).
Misuse	The term 'misuse' should be applied to use that is unlawful (illegal or illicit), or which is not socially or medically

approved, and which has the potential to cause harm. The term 'hazardous use' is also applied to potentially harmful use.

Harmful use   This term should follow the ICD–10 definition, that 'there must be clear evidence that the substance use was responsible for or substantially contributed to physical or psychological harm' (World Health Organization, 1992). 'Problematic use' is an alternative term.

Dependence   The criteria for the diagnosis of dependence are described in Chapter 1. Recent research indicates that a significant minority of young people do develop dependence, especially on alcohol, nicotine, opiates and cannabis. If, unusually, dependence is diagnosed in a young person, this diagnosis has important treatment implications. The term 'addiction' is commonly used to describe 'dependence'.

Interview protocol

Information on the effects of different substances on affect, cognitive function and perception are summarised in Table 10.1. Useful reviews on screening and assessment instruments are available (Crome, 1997; Meyers et al, 1999; Winters et al, 2001). An outline schedule is provided in Table 10.2, and practitioners should think in terms of constructing their own individual schedule for history taking that is appropriate for their situation.

Knowledge of the local drug scene

It is extremely useful to be familiar with the cost and availability of substances in the local area, as there is often considerable variation even within an area.

Almost always the substance problem is not the only problem

It will become obvious almost always that a young person's substance problem is not the only problem, and the assessment should be carried out within this context. It is not too far fetched to suggest that practitioners should assume that this is the case until proven otherwise.

Profile of the young person's vulnerability and resilience

When the young person is predisposed to the consultation, there is a need to establish some of the initial and current reasons for substance use, since they can inform the treatment plan. There are very many reasons, such as recreation, social conformity, mood enhancement or coping with stress. Exploration of the young person's expectations of the negative physical and psychosocial effects and future health concerns, as well as the positive gains (e.g. benefit to social life and mood), will be a further anchor for treatment and assessment of motivation to change.

Readiness to change is another important dimension. To what extent does the young person acknowledge the need to review and alter his or her lifestyle, and how does this affect suitability for treatment? If a 'coercive' approach is being considered, is this a fair decision, or does the young person perceive it as a 'threat' or as the use of 'force'?

An overall general evaluation of the young person's psychological well-being, social involvement with non-drug-using friends, intellectual ability and maturity is helpful in the construction of a profile of capacity to cope and solve problems. Likewise, social support, particularly confidants, provides potential protective factors that can be harnessed in the treatment plan.

Reliability of patient report

Young people are generally more reliable than might be assumed. This information comes from clinical experience and research on collateral information from school and parents, tests of reliability and from 'trick' questions in surveys. These findings also hold true for parental reports.

Cooperation

Cooperation will obviously be hampered if young people are assessed against their will or if they perceive the problem to be non-existent or less severe than does the person making the referral. It is very difficult to make a meaningful assessment if the young person is intoxicated or in withdrawal and, after an evaluation of safety issues, it is usually more sensible to arrange another time (if on an in-patient ward) or appointment.

Developmental stage

The developmental stage, particularly in terms of delay in development, might well affect the young person's perception or report of problems (e.g. exaggeration or underplaying). The assessment techniques used to facilitate disclosure, receptivity to treatment and appreciation of what this might entail are all linked to the developmental stage. The young person may be willing to disclose details of substance use but may be unable to do so, in terms of age, capacity to concentrate and ability to articulate. In this context it should be noted that some young people may choose to manipulate the process by inconsistent, inappropriate and exaggerated responses.

Table 10.1 Symptoms of intoxication and withdrawal

Substance	Intoxication	Withdrawal

Alcohol	Disinhibition
	Argumentativeness
	Aggression
	Interference with personal
	  functioning
	Labile mood
	Impaired judgement and attention
	Unsteady gait and difficulty in
	  standing
	Slurred speech
	Nystagmus
	Decreased level of consciousness
	Flushed face
	Conjunctival injection
		Tremor (tongue, eyelids, hands)
		Agitation, insomnia, malaise
		Convulsions
		Visual, auditory, tactile illusions or
		  hallucinations

Opiates	Apathy
	Sedation, drowsiness, slurred
	  speech
	Disinhibition
	Psychomotor retardation
	Impaired attention and judgement
	Pupillary constriction
	Decreased level of consciousness
	Interference with personal
	  functioning
		Craving
		Sneezing, yawning, runny eyes
		Muscle aches, abdominal pains
		Nausea, vomiting, diarrhoea
		Goose flesh, recurrent chills
		Pupillary dilatation
		Restless sleep

Cannabis	Euphoria and disinhibition
	Anxiety and agitation
	Suspiciousness and paranoid
	  ideation
	Impaired reaction time, judgement
	  and attention
	Hallucinations with preserved
	  orientation
	Depersonalisation and derealisation
	Increased appetite
	Dry mouth
	Conjunctival injection
	Tachycardia
		Anxiety
		Irritability
		Tremor
		Sweating
		Muscle aches

Table continues opposite

Self-efficacy

Assessment of self-efficacy of the young person (i.e. confidence in personal decision-making ability) is imperative because it is predictive of a capacity to choose goals, to expend effort in achieving those goals and to persist in adversity.

Table 10.1 *continued*

Substance	Intoxication	Withdrawal
Nicotine	Craving Malaise or weakness Anxiety, irritability, moodiness Insomnia Increased appetite Increased cough and mouth ulceration Difficulty concentrating Tachycardia and cardiac arrhythmias	Insomnia Bizarre dreams Fluctuating mood Derealisation Interference with personal functioning Nausea Sweating
Stimulants	Euphoria and increased energy Hypervigilance Repetitive stereotyped behaviours Grandiose beliefs and actions Paranoid ideation Abusiveness, aggression and argumentativeness Auditory, tactile and visual hallucinations Sweats, chills, muscular weakness Nausea or vomiting, weight loss Pupillary dilatation, convulsions Tachycardia, arrhythmias, chest pain, hypertension Agitation	Lethargy Psychomotor retardation or agitation Craving Increased appetite Insomnia or hypersomnia Bizarre and unpleasant dreams

Family and educational assessments

Close ties to family and to school tend to inhibit drug use. Conversely, troubled, abusive or absent relationships tend to thrust young people towards deviant peers and substance use. Hence, family and educational assessments are key to understanding the pathway to substance use in younger adolescents.

Seeing the young person with key others facilitates judgements about relationships (e.g. quality of warmth, levels of conflict, trust, degree of supervision). It may be possible to discern to what extent the adults have insight into, influence over and interest in reducing the young person's substance use.

Substance users often have had scholastic problems. These may be due to specific learning disability or persisting attention-deficit hyperactivity disorder. Review of school records, liaison with the school and a thorough history of educational activities and achievement will provide some basis for co-planning realistic educational and vocational rehabilitation for the young person.

Table 10.2 Protocol for history taking

Components of history	Specific details
Demographic characteristics	Age Gender School, college or employment Nationality and religious affiliation Living arrangements – e.g. with parent(s), relatives, friends, homeless, institutional care General environment – e.g. deprivation, affluence, violence
Presenting complaint(s) Each substance should be discussed separately: Alcohol Amphetamines Benzodiazepines Cannabis Cocaine Ecstasy Heroin and other opiates Methadone Nicotine Over-the-counter medication Prescribed medication	May or may not be a substance problem Age of initiation ('first tried') Age of onset of weekend use Age of onset of weekly use Age of onset of daily use Pattern of use during each day Route of use – oral, smoking, snorting, intramuscular, intravenous Age of onset of specific withdrawal symptoms and features of dependence syndrome Current use over previous day, week, month Current cost of use Maximum use ever How is the substance use being funded? Periods of abstinence Triggers to relapse Preferred substance(s) and reasons
Treatment episodes for substance problems	Dates, service, practitioner details Treatment interventions, success or otherwise
Family history	Parents, siblings, grandparents, uncles, aunts History of substance misuse and related problems History of psychiatric problems – e.g. suicide, deliberate self-harm, depression, anxiety, psychotic illness History of physical illness Separation, divorce, death Family relationships, conflict, support Occupational history
Medical history	Episodes of acute or chronic illnesses: respiratory, infective, HIV, hepatitis Hospital admission: dates, problems, treatment, outcome
Psychiatric history	Assessment by general practitioner for any 'minor' complaints (e.g. anxiety, depression) Treatment by general practitioner with psychoactive drugs Referral to psychiatric services: dates, diagnosis, treatment and outcome

Table continues opposite

Table 10.2 *Continued*

Components of history	Specific details
Personal history	Developmental milestones
Educational background	Age started and left school School reports Educational psychology reports Achievements and aspirations Truancy Special educational needs Suspension and exclusion
Training and occupational activities	Ongoing activities and plans
Criminal activities	Involvement in criminal activities preceding or directly related to substance problems Cautions, charges, convictions Probation service involvement Shoplifting, violence, prostitution
Social services	Child protection history Child abuse and neglect
Social environment	Level of community support
Social activities	Sports, hobbies, community work, religious affiliation and activities
Financial situation	Debt to finance substance problems
Useful information	Current address Telephone number, including mobile phone General practitioner's name, address and telephone number Details of other professionals involved
Investigations	Biochemical, haematological, urinary Special investigations (e.g. brain scan) Psychometric testing
Collateral information	Family and friends School Social services Criminal justice agencies Health services Voluntary agencies
Consent and confidentiality	

Determining the next step

Mental state examination

A mental state examination should cover any symptoms of withdrawal or intoxication from the substances that the young person has admitted using. The state of alertness or sedation should be noted, as should the state of dress and general demeanour, including recent weight loss. Observations of slurred speech, pupillary constriction or dilatation, facial flushing, anxiety or calmness, motor agitation or slowing, and sweating or chills may indicate whether the young person has recently used or is withdrawing from drugs. Recent injecting sites, bloodshot eyes, nicotine stains on fingers, signs of liver disease, steadiness of gait, blood pressure and tremulousness are further signs that provide hints of the extent of substance use, and these should be specifically examined. Assessment of concentration, attention, and short- and longer-term memory may point to the excessive use of substances. The presence of abnormal perceptual experiences may suggest the use of cannabis, alcohol, amphetamine or cocaine, or a primary psychotic illness. Establishment of the degree of insight and motivation, as well as appraisal of the intellectual level of the young person, is central to designing the treatment strategy. The level of understanding of the risks posed by the behaviour and lifestyle may determine the young person's ability to consent to or refuse treatment.

Further investigations

It is almost always worthwhile to do some preliminary biochemical and haematological investigations and urine analysis, since these may provide corroborating evidence of the clinical picture (Drummond & Ghodse, 1999; Wolff *et al*, 1999). The practitioner should be certain that the body fluids (blood, urine, saliva) sent for investigation genuinely are the young person's. It is now possible to do mouth swabs, which are less intrusive than other investigations. Most substances are detectable for a few days only. Some longer-acting medications or substances (e.g. benzodiazepines, cannabis, methadone) may be detected some weeks after administration. If a substance is not present, this does not necessarily indicate that a young person is not using it, and the tests should be repeated. If substance misusers are severely dependent, it very unlikely that substances will not be detected. Thus if there are repeated negative results for someone otherwise believed to be dependent, the history has to be questioned. Young people do sometimes exaggerate the amount that they are using: only if there is evidence that drugs are repeatedly being used should, for example, substitution medication be prescribed.

Immediate admission

It may be necessary to arrange for admission or accommodation – very occasionally immediately – in certain cases. These cases would typically involve severe and chaotic substance misuse, deliberate self-harm or suicidal ideation, intravenous use with complications, social isolation, homelessness, abuse and repeated failed community detoxification.

Conclusion

The review of the nature and extent of substance misuse and related problems, and decisions on further management, must be made on the clinician's balanced interpretation of the systematic history, the clinical condition on presentation and the results of physical investigations. Once a particular phase of the consultation is complete, it is important to communicate the formulation of the assessment to the young person, the family and to relevant professionals, for further consultation and action.

References

Crome, I. B. (1997) Editorial. Young people and substance problems – from image to imagination. *Drugs: Education, Prevention and Policy*, **4**, 107–116.

Department of Health (1999) *Drug Misuse and Dependence – Guidelines on Clinical Management*. Norwich: The Stationery Office.

Drummond, C. & Ghodse, H. (1999) Use of investigations in the diagnosis and management of alcohol disorders. *Advances in Psychiatric Treatments*, **5**, 366–375.

Edwards, G., Marshall, E. J. & Cook, C. C. H. (1997) *The Treatment of Drinking Problems*. Cambridge: Cambridge University Press.

Farrell, M., Crome, I. B. & Strang, J. (eds) (1996) Section 28: alcohol- and drug-related problems. In *Oxford Textbook of Medicine* (eds D. J. Weatherall, J. G. G. Ledingham & D. A. Warrell), pp. 4263–4304. Oxford: Oxford University Press.

Ghodse, A. H. (1995) *Drugs and Addictive Behaviour: A Guide to Treatment* (2nd edn). Oxford: Blackwell Science.

Glass, I. B., Farrell, M. & Hajek, P. (1991) Tell me about the client: history taking and formulating cases. In *International Handbook of Addiction Behaviour* (ed. I. B. Glass), pp. 186–191. London: Routledge.

Meyers, K., Hagan, T. A., Zanis, D., *et al* (1999) Critical issues in adolescent substance use assessment. *Drug and Alcohol Dependence*, **55**, 235–246.

Winters, K. C., Latimer, W. W. & Stinchfield, R. (2001) Assessing adolescent substance misuse. In *Innovations in Adolescent Substance Abuse Interventions* (eds E. F. Wagner & H. Waldron), pp. 1–30. Amsterdam: Pergamon Press.

Wolff, K., Welch, S. & Strang, J. (1999) Specific laboratory investigations for assessments and management of drug problems. *Advances in Psychiatric Treatment*, **5**, 180–191.

World Health Organization (1992) *ICD–10 Classification of Mental and Behavioural Disorders*. Geneva: World Health Organization.

CHAPTER 11

Treatment

Ilana B. Crome, Paul McArdle, Eilish Gilvarry and Sue Bailey

Key points

- The multiple individual and developmental needs of young people who use substances need to be recognised by clinicians who provide services for them.
- Substance misuse in young people is a result of complex dysfunction between the young person and the family, school and environment.
- The interventions provided interact with the familial, cultural and environmental background of the young person.
- Treatment should follow a comprehensive assessment and be part of an overall management plan, adapted to the intensity and complexity of the presenting problems.
- Emphasis must be placed on engagement and retention in services.
- Collaborative working with other professionals based on a broadly based multi-component approach is essential.
- Current treatment approaches use or adapt evidence-based techniques, where available, from the adult addiction as well as the child and adolescent mental health fields.
- Cognitive and behavioural approaches, family-based approaches, motivational enhancement and relapse prevention therapies have empirical support from the adult literature and have much in common with other cognitive–behavioural therapies for young people with behavioural problems.
- Overall, the evidence indicates that treatment is effective, but since young substance misusers are heterogeneous, no single approach is universally effective.

Introduction

The demand for treatment of substance misuse has grown. Indeed, many adult addiction services, and to a lesser extent child and adolescent mental health services, have attempted to react positively and rapidly to meet this developing need. Little regard has been paid to evaluating the effectiveness of these programmes, explicitly with reference to young people.

This chapter first examines the effectiveness of a variety of treatment programmes and specific interventions. The psychological and pharmacological modalities for the treatment of substance misuse and psychiatric comorbidity are then described.

Any service offering treatment needs to recognise the different individual and developmental needs of the young person. Adolescence may be conceptualised as a sensitive period, during which 'psychological functions may mature more readily if the right conditions are present' (Rutter & Rutter, 1993). Consequently, failure to address adolescent drug use and related problems can delay or frustrate the adolescent's capacity to assume behaviours critical to responsible adulthood (Hser *et al*, 2001).

Interventions should follow a comprehensive assessment and be part of an overall care and management plan, adapted to the intensity and complexity of the presenting problems. Such a 'stepped care' approach may range from assisting the adolescent's personal efforts to change, without formal treatment but with simple information and advice, to parental and family support and guidance. Treatment should use or adapt evidence-based techniques from the adult addiction and the child and adolescent mental health fields.

Also, those who work with troubled young people must have professional experience of their needs, or be able to work collaboratively with those who do. It is crucial that treatment facilities, while able to respond to relatively uncomplicated or transient difficulties, should also be able to recognise and address the complexities and the comorbidities of the most troubled groups. Overall management plans must take into account aspects such as educational needs, family attachments, physical and psychological health and any likely child protection concerns. Lifestyle issues, including sexuality, as well as general health factors, peer relationships and psychological distress, are all part of the picture.

Since substance misuse in children or adolescents is most usefully viewed as a symptom of complex dysfunction in the young person and the family, school and environment, rather than a 'disease', a broadly based multi-component approach is essential. In addition, as an intervention will affect the familial, cultural and educational backgrounds of the child or adolescent, an interactive dynamic involving that total environment ensues.

Faced with this complexity, many child health or mental health practitioners will be inclined to refer a young person with a substance misuse problem to a specialist service before they institute treatment for the 'underlying disorder' (Crome, 1999; Riggs *et al*, 1999). However, it is often difficult to engage these young people even once – hence multiple referrals are not desirable. Furthermore, treatment of the underlying disorder may play a critical part in the reduction of substance misuse. Since it is important that practitioners are able to assess and intervene in a holistic way, a range of interventions are described below, many of which have applicability to the generalist.

The evidence that treatment works

Evaluation of treatment programmes

There have been only two descriptive outcome studies on adolescent substance misuse in the UK. One has been on adolescent alcohol dependence, the other on young heroin-dependent people treated with methadone by an innovative community service (Doyle *et al*, 1994; Crome *et al*, 1998, 2000). Initial indications are that, despite their multiple disadvantages, the majority of these young people were retained in treatment. The young heroin misusers demonstrated different degrees of success in multiple outcome domains (psychosocial functioning, substance misuse, physical health, methadone reduction) over a range of follow-up periods. However, a sizeable minority, 40%, made substantial improvements on psychosocial functioning, including attainment and maintenance of abstinence.

Much more work has been carried out in the United States. However, in the studies evaluated there were a range of methodological problems, such as little standardisation in assessment of substance use, misuse and dependence; self-report as the major source of information; and inconsistency in the information elicited regarding social, educational and familial background.

There have been few well-controlled studies of specific treatments for adolescent substance misuse. Catalano *et al* (1990) reviewed 29 treatment outcome studies. Although many of these studies had design flaws, the authors concluded that 'some treatment' was superior to 'no treatment'. They also concluded that there was little evidence to suggest that particular modalities were more effective and that conclusive controlled studies had not been undertaken. Factors for success included staff characteristics, the availability of special services and family participation. Length of treatment was related to reduced alcohol and drug misuse in residential treatment programmes. Characteristics that predicted poor compliance were younger age of onset, serious alcohol misuse, use of multiple drugs and severity of behavioural disorder. Predictors of relapse included cravings for alcohol, low involvement in work, and little involvement in hobbies and other leisure activities.

A review by Williams & Chang (2000) reviewed outcome studies of eight multi-programme, multi-site interventions and 45 single-programme interventions for adolescent substance misuse. In the eight studies that reported on abstinence, the average sustained abstinence rate at six months was 38% and at 12 months 32%. Furthermore, 66.6% of relapses occurred in the first three months after treatment. Although only a minority of adolescents actually achieved abstinence by the end of treatment, reduction in substance use was reported in 12 of the 13 studies in which this was measured. There were some reports of a 50–60% reduction in substance use at discharge or at one-year follow-up and the majority (12) of studies demonstrated some reduction. Of the eight studies in which these were evaluated, an effect of treatment on illegal behaviour was reported by five, on mental health by four, on family problems by three, and on school functioning by three. Thus, the majority of adolescents who enter treatment improve in terms of substance use and general functioning, but in view of the lack of treatment control groups, it is not possible to know whether this could be attributed to natural recovery. In the 15 studies that compared treatments, nine demonstrated the advantage of one treatment over another.

Hser *et al* (2001) evaluated drug treatments for 1167 adolescents in four cities in the United States. A naturalistic non-experimental design was used. Consecutive adolescent admissions to 23 community-based teams were studied from 1993 to 1995. This included admissions to short- and long-term in-patient units and out-patient programmes. This confirmed the profile of adolescents with multiple problems – for example, 58% of patients were involved with the legal system and 63% met criteria for mental disorder. The multi-modal interventions included group work, family therapy and individual therapeutic sessions (rather like on adolescent day or in-patient psychiatric units). In the year following treatment, cannabis use was halved from 80% to 44%, and heavy drinking was reduced from 33% to 20%. Illicit drug use was reduced from 48% to 42%, and criminal justice involvement from 75% to 53%. In addition, psychosocial functioning improved. Thus, planned comparisons of different intervention programmes also reveal important reductions in substance use, and criminality, and improvement in well-being. These effects occurred irrespective of whether there was a residential component to the intervention. Again, after controlling for the initial severity of the problem, length of intervention was positively associated with outcome. This is consistent with the view of clinicians and researchers in the child and adolescent mental health, adult addiction and prevention fields that many of these young people have vulnerabilities that persist or recur. Hence, long-term follow-up and booster sessions are required for optimal outcome.

Brown *et al* (2001) assessed four-year outcomes from an adolescent drug and alcohol treatment centre, which adopted the 12-step approach to abstinence. (The '12-step' approach is derived from the abstinence philosophy and peer-support approach of Alcoholics Anonymous/ Narcotics Anonymous.) The findings are striking. First, while the greatest reduction was found in stimulant use, and there was some reduction in alcohol and marijuana use, nicotine use continued in 75% of patients. Secondly, five groups of young people were described: abstainers (7%), users (8%), slow improvers (8%), worse with time (25%), and continuous heavy users (48%). This points to substantial diversity of outcome. Not surprisingly, better functioning in multiple domains was found in abstainers compared with 'worse with time' and 'heavy users'. Thirdly, despite improvement, this group demonstrated greater use than in the general population. The authors underlined the need for more research and for enhanced provision in terms of duration, types of psychosocial support and specific treatment interventions and settings. Undoubtedly, the scarcity of designated programmes for substance-misusing teenagers is partially responsible for the lack of evidence.

Evaluation of individual approaches

Information-based methods

There is considerable evidence from other health and social care fields that an information-based approach has useful effects when the information is given in non-complex presentations (Powell *et al*, 2001). Peer support and advice is a further low-cost intervention that has proven useful in similar situations (Shah *et al*, 2001). While there are counter-arguments, especially concerning 'contagion', peer support may have a role in the management of substance problems in schools and other youth-oriented environments. There is still a need to evaluate these approaches further with substance-using young people in, for instance, primary care (tier 1) settings. If they are as useful as in related fields, then primary care staff could respond constructively to the queries that may present at that level.

Brief, minimal or short-term interventions

The idea that most adult substance misusers do not require lengthy interventions has been the pivotal conceptual shift that has influenced service delivery over the past 20 years (Bien *et al*, 1993; Dunn *et al*, 2001; Wutzke *et al*, 2002). Here the term 'brief' is used interchangeably with 'minimal' and 'short-term' intervention, since these types of treatments are partly distinguished by their relative brevity, delivery by a non-specialist, sometimes opportunistically, on a one-to-one basis in an out-patient or community setting. The administration of a screening tool (e.g. the AUDIT questionnaire; Saunders *et al*, 1993) sometimes precedes the intervention, when it may be aimed at those excessive drinkers with goals of moderate consumption rather than abstinence. The advice given is brief, non-judgemental, personalised if possible, and supported by self-help materials. For example, a primary care worker may suggest that 'smoking is not good for your health', or say 'have a look at your liver test results, which indicate that you are damaging your liver by drinking'. The term may also refer to an hour-long session of motivational interviewing, or six sessions of cognitive–behavioural treatment, delivered by specialised practitioners, whereas longer-term intensive interventions are typically delivered in an in-patient or residential setting and are provided by a specialist team.

There is good evidence of the effectiveness, and cost-effectiveness, of these interventions with alcohol misusers in primary care settings, in accident and emergency departments and in educational settings (Longabaugh *et al*, 2001). This type of approach has also proven effective with cigarette smoking (Richmond & Anderson, 1994). Research from the United States and Australia on the use of these interventions with young people has produced some promising results (Senft *et al*, 1997; Aubrey, 1998; Monti *et al*, 1999; Hulse *et al*, 2001). Even if the success rates are relatively modest, if widely and consistently applied there could be gains to public health.

Psychological and pharmacological modalities

Deas & Thomas (2001) provide an overview of ten controlled studies conducted since 1990. These studies evaluated family behaviour therapy and individual cognitive–behavioural therapy (CBT) as well as pharmacological interventions and 12-step approaches. CBT, on the other hand, focuses on thoughts, beliefs, attitudes and assumptions that might impede behaviour change. It should be noted that sample sizes were small, ranging from 10 to 135, with half having fewer than 26 participants. The age range, baseline and follow-up assessments were variable. The findings did not consistently indicate the superiority of particular modalities, though there appeared to be a trend indicating the effectiveness of individual behavioural and family therapy. When sertraline and CBT were compared with placebo and CBT, both groups demonstrated reductions in substance use (Deas-Nesmith *et al*, 1998). Also, when 12-step therapy was compared with CBT, alcohol reduction was evident with 12-step treatment, but there were no other differences. Myers *et al* (1993) recruited 80 teenagers admitted to in-patient adolescent drug and alcohol programmes: problem-focused coping predicted less use of drugs and alcohol at follow-up. Two other studies examined behavioural therapy (Azrin *et al*, 1994; Kaminer *et al*, 1998) and showed improvement in drug use, as well as school and work attendance and behaviour.

Evaluation of family therapies

There are a variety of family therapies, but they have much in common and broadly similar goals. Family therapy approaches have received most attention in clinical research on treatment for adolescents with substance misuse. When evaluated in relation to their differential effect on children with disruptive behaviour, their effect sizes are similar (Barkley *et al*, 1992). In a meta-analysis, Stanton & Shadish (1997) found support for the superiority of family therapy (but not family education or support) for adolescent substance use disorders over other modalities. Joanning *et al* (1992) conducted a pre-test/post-test comparison of three models of adolescent drug misuse treatment: family systems therapy, adolescent group therapy and family drug education. Family systems therapy was superior. One commonly used model is structural strategic family therapy (Szapocznik *et al*, 1989).

In a sense, these findings substantiated older studies of multi-modal interventions which addressed complex behaviour disorder such as conduct disorder, but which did not always explicitly target drug misuse. They provided potentially important clues to successful intervention. For instance, Satterfield *et al* (1987) compared the long-term outcome for children with behaviour disorder following a drug-only condition (methylphenidate) with those following a combined drug and multi-modal treatment. The latter was designed to provide a range of interventions, including individual CBT, educational and group therapies, sustained over a two- to three-year period. They reported significantly reduced arrest and institutionalisation rates among those with extended multi-modal treatment compared with those receiving the drug-only intervention. The effect of a shorter-term multi-modal treatment was between that of the drug-only and of the extended (two- to three-year) multi-modal interventions.

Multi-systemic therapy

Two multi-modal forms of family therapy have been evaluated specifically in relation to substance misuse. Both multi-dimensional family therapy (MDFT) and multi-systemic therapy (MST) are adaptations of family therapy. As well as classical family therapy goals, they aim to address determinants of substance misuse, including peer influences, that are external to the family. Schmidt *et al* (1996) found substantial improvements in parenting after MDFT. Randomised trials have demonstrated the effectiveness of both in the management of young people's substance problems (Henggeler *et al*, 1998, 1999; Liddle *et al*, 2001). The findings support the view that a substantial reduction in substance misuse may parallel improvements in family relationships, enhanced diversionary activities and affiliation with non-using peer groups.

In a randomised trial funded by the National Institute on Drug Abuse (NIDA), the effectiveness of MST was measured with juvenile offenders who met criteria for substance abuse or dependence, according to DSM–III–R (American Psychiatric Association, 1987) (Henggeler *et al*, 1998). Early findings suggest that the application of MST led to a significant decrease in drug use. MST reduced re-arrests by 26% in comparison with usual services, although this figure was not statistically significant. At one year after referral, MST had reduced days incarcerated by 46% and total days in out-of-home placement by 50%. MST has the capacity to address a long-standing problem in the field of substance misuse treatment, namely high drop-out rates. In the studies, 98% of the families in the MST condition completed a full course of treatment, which lasted on average 130 days.

Therapy takes place predominantly in the young person's home. It is thought that the minimisation of drop-out is due to the following key elements of the MST approach:

- Therapists are available 24 hours a day, 7 days a week.
- The MST treatment team and project administrators assume responsibility for achieving treatment, engagement and clinical outcome.
- Treatment is strength focused and goals are set primarily by family members.
- Services are individualised to meet the multiple and changing needs of youths and their families.

Thus, by providing services that were accessible, fully collaborative and emphasised family strengths, treatment was provided in full to almost all families.

Great concern has been expressed about mental health, juvenile justice and substance misuse services for young people, and undoubtedly tremendous resources are being spent in these areas, but demonstrated effectiveness is more difficult to establish (McGuire & Priestley, 1995). It should be noted that most of the evaluations of these therapies have been conducted in the United States, in well-resourced settings that are not always matched by the realities of clinical practice in the UK. Indeed, one of the distinctive features of MST is its intensity: it requires case-loads of perhaps three individuals and almost daily supervision sessions (Henggeler *et al*, 1999), which are virtually unknown in UK community-based practice. The only exception is those children who are in residential care or in child and adolescent mental health day or in-patient units. For this reason, it may best be regarded as a potential alternative to residential interventions.

A further valid criticism of the work undertaken, particularly in the effectiveness evaluation and cost evaluation of MST, is that much of it has been carried out by the team itself.

There are also the inherent risks of rolling out very specialist training in different cultures and different countries. The critical issue is whether work that is carried out by teams that are distal to the birthplace of any treatment development can and does deliver MST with the same level of integrity needed to obtain the demonstrated clinical outcomes. A vital task, then, is to evaluate those factors that are linked to treatment adherence. Early indications are that high-cost, low-routine service delivery has to be targeted at those with the most severe levels of offending. However, there are currently MST projects being carried out in Canada, where the research evaluation is being done out by the Canadian government (Leschied & Cunningham, 2002, personal communication).

In a study of mental health treatment, substance misuse treatment and out-of-home placement, the incremental costs of MST (i.e. the costs of MST that were above and beyond the usual cost of services for these young people) were shown to be nearly offset by the savings incurred as a result of reduction in days in out-of-home placements (i.e. incarceration and residential in-patient treatment) during the first year (Schoenwald *et al*, 1996). Thus, while resource intensive, MST may be an alternative to, and more economically acceptable than, residential treatments. The main proponents of this therapy argue that it poses challenges to policy makers and providers: the emphasis is on providers to engage and retain families, a need for enhanced skills and competence and, where there is reliance on residential services, appropriate shifts in resources.

Multi-component behaviour therapy

The treatment theory underlying multi-component behaviour therapy (MBT) is based on a behavioural understanding of drug dependence, and conceptualises drug use as being reinforced by both the pharmacological effects of the drug itself (i.e. 'the high') and contingencies in the user's ecology (e.g. family, vocational, educational, social and recreational) that support drug use and discourage abstinence. This conceptualisation has significant empirical support (Higgins *et al*, 1994) and differs from other perspectives on drug dependence, such as disease, self-medication and moral models.

Evaluation of group therapies

In evaluating group therapy, care should be taken in the selection of the membership. This is because groups composed solely of substance misusers may propagate misuse. However, groups can be a useful component of interventions. This positive view is derived from the evaluation of group therapy. The impact of school-based groups in particular has been evaluated in the UK and proved particularly valuable in sustained improvement in general social and behavioural adjustment (Kolvin *et al*, 1981; McArdle *et al*, 2002), but they have not been evaluated with substance use as an outcome variable.

While individual adult 12-step therapy, CBT and motivational enhancement therapy have empirical support (Project MATCH Research Group, 1997*a,b*), there is limited evidence of effectiveness in groups. An abstinence goal may deter engagement and retention of the most complex vulnerable young people, with whom the lesser goal of harm reduction might produce health gains.

Kaminer *et al* (1998; Kaminer & Burleson, 1999) randomised dually diagnosed adolescent substance misusers into two 12-week manual guided out-patient group psychotherapies: CBT and interactional treatment (IT). Although it was hypothesised that patients with externalising disorders would fare better with CBT, and those with internalising disorders with IT, at three months no matching effects were found. Adolescents assigned to CBT demonstrated significant reduction in severity of substance use compared with those assigned to IT. School function, peer relationships, legal problems and psychiatric severity demonstrated consistent non-significant improvements with CBT over IT. At 15-month follow-up no further improvements were evident but initial gains were maintained. This was interpreted as being a promising short-term psychosocial intervention for adolescents. It was suggested that larger, longer-term randomised controlled studies are required to examine treatment interventions.

Costs of interventions

A further examination of treatment of comorbid conditions relates to that of cost-effectiveness. King *et al* (2000) described the co-occurrence of psychiatric and substance use diagnoses in adolescents in different service systems. The frequency, severity, recognition, costs and outcomes were analysed in this, the Fort Bragg Demonstration Project. In a sample of 428 adolescents, providers' diagnoses were compared with the researchers' diagnoses. Only 21 of 59 cases with comorbid conditions were identified by providers. Not surprisingly, there were differences between services in recognition, but not frequency or severity of cases. Comorbid clients had more behavioural problems and more impairment of functioning, and treatment costs were more than twice ($30,000) those of non-comorbid cases ($13,000). However, mental health outcomes were *not* influenced by the type of service system, comorbid diagnosis, or treatment. Screening and treatment of substance misuse is potentially cost saving in mental health and other services treating young people (O'Brien, 1997).

149

Descriptive outline of psychological modalities used in practice

The aim of this and the following section (on pharmacological modalities) is not only to describe the techniques, but also to indicate the contexts in which they are translated into the therapeutic tools required by those assisting young substance misusers.

The role of non-traditional treatment pathways to recovery, as well as the diversity and intensity of psychological techniques in the spectrum of treatment settings, needs to be identified and if relevant, incorporated. It is important to attempt to discriminate between natural changes, maturation and curative mechanisms. Some young people who use drugs and alcohol – sometimes problematically and in high-risk situations – may gradually, or even abruptly, cease use. This resilience or potential for 'natural recovery' may be explained by strengths in the individual or the family, or other environmental influences. A good therapist, sensitive to nuances in actions and behaviour, will take advantage of personal strengths, protective factors, favourable opportunities or positive events in the life of the young person. Such understanding may be a substitute for formal treatment. It relies on a feel for and knowledge of the development of the young, and comes with training and experience.

Informed by a detailed assessment, the clinician's role may be to educate and to reassure. While potentially useful tools in the treatment repertoire, they should be used with a clear understanding of their limitations. It is essential that information is accurate, up to date and is made readily available to both young people and their families. The choice of language, both in terms of the literacy skills required and the attractiveness and appropriateness to young people, is of the essence. It should relate to the diversity of languages and colloquialisms that may be in use. Information for parents and carers is vital in order to allow them to converse with young people, to understand the terms used, to reduce and reframe their anxieties and so improve communication with the young. Use of the internet, in particular local websites designed by young people, may be a valuable resource. However, these should be screened for misinformation. Accurate guidance must not only address abstinence, but also provide advice and information on responses to intoxication, harm reduction strategies in clubs, warnings about overdose, and sexual and physical health.

Counselling

'Counselling' is a widely used term in the adult literature. It is a form of therapy or intervention that can represent a wide range of theoretical models. There are many different definitions, each emphasising specific aspects of the counselling role and processes practised in a multiplicity of settings. It embodies psychodynamics as well as cognitive–behavioural and person-centred approaches.

The important objectives include:

*   problem solving – developing competence in dealing with a specific problem;
*   acquisition of social skills – mastery of social and interpersonal skills by assertiveness or anger control;
*   cognitive change – modification of irrational beliefs and maladaptive patterns of thought;
*   behaviour change – modification of maladaptive behaviour;
*   systemic change – introducing change into family systems.

We use the term 'counselling' to incorporate brief or intensive interventions, be they supportive, directive or motivational in nature, individual, family or group behavioural treatments, or social network behavioural therapies. Counselling may aim to reduce the use of alcohol and drugs, as well as the negative consequences or related problems (e.g. lifestyle issues such as housing, sexual health or careers).

Counselling may encompass assessment, engagement and support, together with the development of therapeutic relationships. The non-judgemental and empathic method of challenging decisions and assumptions in motivational interviewing is included in the gamut of techniques. It may cover self-monitoring, advice and problem-solving techniques, which include relapse prevention. Wagner *et al* (1999) outlined the components of counselling: information, identification of problems and self-monitoring, recognition of high-risk behaviours, family conflict resolution, the development of social supports and alternatives to substance use, coping strategies and advice on relationships. However, while it is a widely used term, it is imprecise and should not be used without description of objectives and techniques.

From individual therapies to family therapies

Individual approaches to treatment have been based mostly on cognitive–behavioural principles. By identifying and modifying maladaptive thinking patterns, adolescents can reduce their negative thoughts and abusive behaviour, including substance use. In structural strategic family therapy, treatments involve all family members, whether present or not at the sessions, because substance misuse is understood as being related to family dysfunction. Common patterns of family dysfunction targeted in the sessions include under- or over-involvement, avoidance of conflict and insufficient supervision. Family therapy is often accompanied by skills training for the parents. Such approaches aim to reduce the adolescent's substance misuse by changing the parents' management practices.

Effective treatment of complex, multi-determined problems such as substance misuse and antisocial behaviour requires a theoretical basis that will encompass both general systems theory and the theory of social ecology, rather than individual approaches. Taking a systemic view, the whole is considered to represent more than the sum of its parts, and the larger picture is taken into consideration (Pliz, 1992). The social ecologist would propose that the individual's behaviour is influenced by numerous contexts, not all of which are direct, one-to-one interactions. The basic assumption is that behaviour can be fully understood only when it is viewed within naturally occurring contexts. Economic difficulties, the portrayal of violence in the media and prejudice are potential distal influences on a child's behaviour. Treatment specification is a critical task in the development, validation and dissemination of a theoretical approach. For some intervention models, this is relatively easy to specify: for example, behavioural parent training can occur through ten sessions, with well-defined tasks targeted in each session. In contrast, complex, multi-faceted comprehensive and individualised treatments can be difficult to operationalise and specify.

In the field of brief family therapy, Piercy (1986) developed a treatment manual that used 'treatment principles' to guide therapist behaviour. These principles organise therapists' case conceptionalisation, prioritisation of interventions and the type of interventions delivered.

Providing a flexible treatment protocol within the limits of adhering to treatment principles allows therapists the freedom to use any strengths to the family's advantage. The treatment principles can be readily and conveniently used for assisting the ongoing conceptionalisation and design of an intervention. Treatment integrity can be evaluated by measuring therapists' adherence to the principles. These, in turn, have predicted long-term outcomes regarding the criminal activity and incarceration of violent and chronic juvenile offenders who misuse substances (Henggeler *et al*, 1997).

Multi-systemic therapy

Multi-systemic therapy 'can be viewed as a package of interventions that are deployed with children and their families and which focuses on the multiple systems (family, school, peers, neighbourhood) which impact on the child or young person' (Kazdin, 2001). It is a more comprehensive approach than other family therapies. At its core is a family-based treatment approach that uses techniques familiar to family therapists, such as 'joining, reframing, enactment, paradox and assigning specific tasks', as well as techniques derived from behaviour therapy, such as problem-solving skills training. It also recognises that other groupings, such as peers and the school, are crucial and require parallel intervention, 'employing indigenous community resources' (Henggeler *et al*, 1999).

The goal of MST assessment is to 'make sense' of behavioural problems in light of their systemic context, consistent with social ecological models of behaviour and research on the known determinants of antisocial behaviour. MST assessment focuses on understanding the factors that contribute directly or indirectly to behavioural problems. In general, these involve transactions between the child and the multiple systems in which he or she is embedded (i.e. family, peers, school and neighbourhood), as well as transactions between these systems (e.g. family–school interface, family–peer interface).

The MST therapist attempts to determine how each factor, singly or in combination with others, increases or decreases the probability of youth problem behaviours. Several steps are required to develop a comprehensive understanding of a 'fit'.

The principles of MST can be summarised as follows:

- The primary purpose of assessment is to understand the 'fit' between the identified problem and the broader systemic context.
- Therapeutic contact emphasises the positive and uses systemic strengths as levers for change.
- Interventions are designed to promote responsible behaviour and decrease irresponsible behaviour among family members.
- Interventions are focused and action oriented, targeting specific and well-defined problems.
- Interventions target sequences of behaviour within and between multiple systems that maintain the identified problem.
- Interventions are developmentally appropriate to the needs of the youth.
- Interventions are designed to require daily or weekly effort by family members.
- Intervention effectiveness is evaluated continuously from multiple perspectives, with providers assuming responsibility for overcoming barriers.

Interventions are designed to promote treatment generalisation and long-term maintenance of therapeutic change, by empowering carers to address family members' needs. Nevertheless, some services are reluctant to engage parents because of issues of confidentiality and fears of reduced engagement with the young person. Clearly, the extent of involvement will depend on the nature of the problem and the age of the child. However, the empirical findings, which are consistent with the experience of child and adolescent mental health services, underscore the importance of working with families.

Multi-component behaviour therapy

Like MST, MBT interventions are individualised, focused on the present, and target well-defined problems with behavioural and ecological interventions. An individualised treatment plan is based on a functional analysis of the young person's substance misuse. The young person is taught to identify all stimuli or 'triggers' – people, places, time of day, smells, sights, sounds, activities, moods, thoughts – that lead to and reinforce substance use. Using this information the triggers (e.g. the car of a friend who also uses), the drug-using behaviour (e.g. the snorting of cocaine), the positive consequences of use (e.g. feeling the usual short-term exuberance of the drug use) and the negative (usually longer-term) consequences of use (e.g. financial relationship disharmonies) are identified. This information is then used to design individualised interventions to restructure the young person's ecology in order to eliminate or reduce exposure to ecological triggers and change self-statements and beliefs that serve as triggers (e.g. 'I can't go on', 'I can't make it without a hit'). The lifestyle changes have to incorporate activities engaging and reinforcing enough to compete with the powerful reinforcing effects of drug use; this is the major challenge of the treatment modality. Such lifestyle changes are composed in reality of many small steps, which are taught by the therapist, practised with the therapist and then practised in real-world settings. Another essential ingredient of this form of therapy is that it is actively supported by 'a significant other' who collaborates in treatment. Throughout the treatment process, provision for the swift detection of substance use via monitoring of urine analysis is necessary and needs to be coupled with immediate dispensation of concrete social reinforcers or the withdrawal of such reinforcers.

Group therapies

Participation in self-help groups is an important feature of many treatment programmes. Meetings are often held on treatment units to expose patients to the self-help group process. Community meetings can also facilitate the patient's transfer from the core programme to after-care or follow-up. Adolescents attending these groups receive support from recovering peers and older members. Peers remind the adolescent of the negative consequences of substance misuse.

The 12-step approach is a variant of the self-help group. Central to the 12-steps philosophy is the idea that recovery from addiction is possible only if the individual recognises the problem, and admits that he or she is unable to use substances in moderation.

Residential treatments, such as therapeutic communities, offer long-term intensive psychological interventions. These have typically been used in the United States for people with substance misuse and related problems who require treatment that is intensive, highly structured and of long duration. The communities have been adapted somewhat for adolescents, with shorter stays, less confrontation, more adult supervision, more emphasis on education, and enhancement of family involvement. The relatively few studies that have been undertaken have reported that long-term residential treatments are more effective than out-patient modalities, with length of stay crucial. The most consistent outcome is that of improvement in criminal involvement.

Pharmacological agents

General issues

Many young people using substances have conditions that can be ameliorated by pharmacological means, occasionally as the main intervention and almost always as an adjunct to psychosocial interventions (Department of Health, 1999). Medication should be used as part of a comprehensive plan that incorporates a variety of individual interventions (e.g. education, psychotherapies) designed to meet the needs of the young person.

The pharmacological management of young substance misusers poses considerable difficulties. First, apart from nicotine replacement therapy (National Institute for Clinical Excellence, 2002) and buprenorphine medications used for detoxification, the use of pharmacological agents for substitution or relapse prevention have not been licensed for use, and are not recommended for use, in anyone under 18 years old. There are few empirical data concerning their use in this age group. It should also be noted that, in the *British National Formulary*, the term 'child' covers patients under 12 years old.

Emergency procedures

Since both opiates and benzodiazepines have specific pharmacological antagonists, naloxone and flumazenil respectively, these are useful in emergencies. General practitioners and paramedics should have naloxone available.

Detoxification

The majority of adolescents are not dependent and so do not generally require detoxification (Stewart & Brown, 1995). Some symptomatic treatment may be useful if there are mild withdrawal symptoms. If detoxification is required, then the same principles apply as for adults. However, particular thought should be given to dosage (depending on the person's body size and age) and awareness of the possibility of misuse (e.g. benzodiazepines).

There are a variety of pharmacological agents that may be helpful in detoxification, but their effectiveness in the detoxification of young people has not been researched. Also, without additional psychological and social support, sustained effectiveness is likely to be limited. In-patient detoxification is quicker and more effective than in the community, but community detoxification is far more widespread. Very few appropriate in-patient (tier 4) facilities exist for adolescent addicts, despite the fact that some of those attending have severe dependence, which requires medically supervised detoxification. Negotiated collaboration with adult addiction, maternity, adolescent mental health and paediatric in-patient units is required to detoxify patients appropriately and safely.

The drugs used for opiate detoxification include methadone, lofexidine, clonidine, buprenorphine and dihydrocodeine. Chlordiazepoxide in the short term is the usual treatment of choice for detoxification in alcohol dependence. Vitamin supplementation during out-patient and in-patient alcohol detoxification should be carefully planned.

Stabilisation/maintenance and reduction

Stabilisation and reduction with methadone take longer with adolescents than with adults, and patient retention in treatment is a key consideration. There is a small but significant number of injecting dependent heroin users presenting to services in England who require intervention and who have derived benefit from methadone stabilisation and slow reduction (Crome *et al*, 2000).

The National Institute for Clinical Excellence (2002) has recommended that young people can receive nicotine replacement therapy (NRT) if prescribed by a medical practitioner.

Paradoxically, the controlled research evidence for the most effective intervention for opiate dependence in adults is for methadone maintenance treatment. There is no research on maintenance in young people. Also, anecdotal evidence from clinicians suggests that there is little role for maintenance in the young population.

Relapse prevention

Pharmacological therapies as adjuncts in relapse prevention include disulfiram, acamprosate and naltrexone in alcohol use, naltrexone in opiate users and bupropion in smokers. Since there has been no research on these adjuncts in young people, and no consensus on their application in clinical practice to young people, they should be undertaken only with caution and by specialised services. The use of 'take home' naloxone has not been evaluated in young people and even more exacting vigilance is needed before this can be advocated.

Psychiatric disorders

Substance-misusing young people referred to clinical services will often have complex comorbidity, conduct disorder, attention-deficit hyperactivity disorder and affective symptoms, as well as educational and psychosocial disadvantages. Some will have behaviours suggestive of borderline personality disorder, and a very few will have early-onset psychosis, whether schizophrenic or bipolar.

Children and adolescents may present with depressive and anxiety disorders that require antidepressant medication. Occasionally, children and young people will present to services with adult-type psychotic conditions that require appropriate pharmacological management. However, many of the youths with complex problems have underlying neurocognitive deficits that manifest as an impaired ability to relate and to communicate, and that are linked to marked attentional problems and hyperkinetic behaviours. Some of these conditions require pharmacological treatment in their own right. Furthermore, probably through facilitation of normal adaptive behaviour at home and particularly at school, stimulant treatment is associated with subsequently reduced illicit drug use (Biederman *et al*, 1999).

Assessment may confirm the presence of psychosocial impairment related to a perhaps previously unrecognised or untreated comorbid disorder. Clinicians should then consider the appropriateness of a trial of stimulant medication such as methylphenidate. Due caution is always required when prescribing a controlled substance (Ghodse, 1999). Doing so to someone known to misuse substances is especially problematic, not least because the medication could add to the potential misuse portfolio of the young person. However, if, for instance, it facilitated school attendance and even educational success, then a significant amelioration in misuse might ensue. Clearly, the clinician must ensure that the medication is kept in a safe place and that it is only part of an appropriate management plan (National Institute for Clinical Excellence, 2000). It must be administered appropriately and there must be a responsible person available to ensure its safety. This will require careful follow-up and close liaison with carers and school.

Conclusion: implementation of evidence-based techniques, good practice and towards innovation

In the past decade there have been significant advances in the understanding of adolescent substance misuse and the development of evidence-based techniques. Young users are heterogeneous, no one approach is universally effective, and evaluation of treatment outcome should be multi-dimensional. In the adult literature, not only have cognitive and behavioural approaches, motivational enhancement therapy, relapse prevention therapy and community reinforcement approaches empirical support, but they have much in common with cognitive–behavioural interventions for children and youths with behaviour problems (Target & Fonagy, 1996). In the child and adolescent substance misuse field, these therapies are just beginning to be systematically studied. Review of other studies of interventions with young people indicates that family therapy adapted to the needs of substance misusers appears to be a useful advance. However, it is acknowledged that the routes to 'natural recovery' are multiple, and require further elucidation. Whatever the treatment label, new friends, success at school or work, emotional support from families, self-help and structured activities are important components.

Where the evidence is lacking, there are a number of good practice principles that must be considered when treating young people with substance misuse (Winters *et al*, 2000; Health Advisory Service, 2001). These should include attention to the unique developmental needs of young people, including delay in normal cognitive and socio-emotional development. While not all young people who use drugs will be dependent, misusers may relapse, and many may have comorbid disorders which must be recognised and treated. Treatment must take into account age, gender, disability, ethnicity, cultural background, and readiness to change. There must be sensitivity to the motivational barriers to change at the outset of treatment, and therapist empathy influences outcome. Family involvement is key and programmes based mainly on adult models are not appropriate.

There is a need for innovation in research specifically directed at young people in the UK. This could include careful descriptive studies, detailed evaluation of ongoing projects, and scrutiny of 'older' techniques in 'newer' settings and situations. Ingenuity may be required in identifying some of the settings where young drinkers or drug users may be found, for it is not only in accident and emergency departments and paediatric wards that the prevalence of substance misuse is high, but also in sexual health clinics, primary care nurses' clinics and generic counselling services. Screening and assessment of these groups of young people, in effect a captive audience, can foster a 'teachable moment' in which to deliver and evaluate brief interventions. Brief interventions must be adapted in form and content to the particular needs of young people, as they may work either alone or, in complex situations, synergistically with other prevention activities, policy measures and specialised treatment interventions. This offers the potential for a significant public health impact in both the short and longer term.

References

American Psychiatric Association (1987) *Diagnostic and Statistical Manual of Mental Disorders* (3rd edn, revised) (DSM–III–R). Washington, DC: American Psychiatric Association.

Aubrey, L. (1998) *Motivational Interviewing with Adolescents Presenting for Outpatient Substance Abuse Treatment.* Doctoral dissertation. University of New Mexico, dissertation abstracts DAI-B 59-03 1357.

Azrin, N. H., Donohue, B., Besalel, V. A., *et al* (1994) Youth drug abuse treatment: a controlled outcome study. *Journal of Child and Adolescent Substance Abuse,* 3, 1–6.

Barkley, R., Guevermont, D., Anastopoulos, A., *et al* (1992) A comparison of three family therapy programs for treating family conflict in adolescents with attention deficit hyperactivity disorder. *Journal of Consulting and Clinical Psychology,* 60, 450–462.

Biederman, J., Wilens, T., Mick, E., *et al* (1999) Pharmacotherapy of attention-deficit/hyperactivity disorder reduces risk of substance use disorder *Paediatrics,* 104, e20.

Bien, T. H., Miller, W. R. & Tonigan, J. S. (1993) Brief interventions for alcohol problems: a review. *Addiction,* 88, 315–336.

Brown, S. A., D'Amico, E. J., McCarthy, D. M., *et al* (2001) Four year outcomes from adolescent alcohol and drug treatment. *Journal of Studies on Alcohol,* 62, 381–388.

Catalano, R. F., Hawkins, J. D., Wells, E. A., *et al* (1990) Evaluation of the effectiveness of adolescent drug abuse treatment, assessment of risks for relapse and promising approaches for relapse prevention. *International Journal of the Addictions,* 25, 1085–1140.

Crome, I. B. (1999) Treatment interventions – looking towards the millennium. *Drug and Alcohol Dependence,* 55, 247–263.

——, Christian, J. & Green, C. (1998) Tip of the national iceberg? Profile of adolescent patients prescribed methadone in an innovative community drug service. *Drugs Education, Prevention and Policy,* 5, 195–197.

——, —— & —— (2000) A unique designated community service for adolescents: policy, prevention and education implications. *Drugs Education, Prevention and Policy,* 7, 87–108.

Deas, D. & Thomas, S. E. (2001) An overview of controlled studies of adolescent substance abuse treatment. *American Journal of Addictions,* 10, 178–189.

Deas-Nesmith, D., Randall, C., Roberts, J., *et al* (1998) Sertraline treatment of depressed adolescent alcoholics: a pilot study. *Alcohol Clinical and Experimental Research,* 22, 74A.

Department of Health (1999) *Guidelines on Clinical Management: Drug Misuse and Dependence.* Norwich: The Stationery Office.

Doyle, H., Delaney, W. & Tobin, J. (1994) Follow-up study of young attenders at an alcohol unit. *Addiction,* 89, 183–189.

Dunn, C., Deroo, L. & Rivara, F. P. (2001) The use of brief interventions adapted from motivational interviewing across behavioural domains: a systematic review. *Addiction,* 96, 1725–1742.

Ghodse, H. (1999) Dramatic increase in methylphenidate consumption. *Current Opinion in Psychiatry,* 12, 265–268.

Health Advisory Service (2001) *The Substance of Young Needs.* London: Drugs Prevention Advisory Service, Home Office.

Henggeler, S. W., Melton, G. B., Brondino, M. J., *et al* (1997) Multi systemic therapy with violent and chronic juvenile offenders and their families: the role of treatment fidelity and successful dissemination. *Journal of Consulting and Clinical Physiology,* 65, 821–833.

——, Borduin, C. M., Melton, G. B., *et al* (1998) Effects of multisystemic therapy on drug use and abuse in serious juvenile offenders: a progress report from two outcome studies. *Family Dynamics of Addiction Quarterly*, **1**, 40–51.

——, Pickeral, S. & Brondino, M. (1999) Multisystemic treatment of substance abusing and dependent delinquents: outcomes, treatment fidelity and transportability. *Mental Health Services Research*, **1**, 171–184.

Higgins, S. T., Budney, A. J. & Bickel, W. K. (1994) Applying behavioural concepts and principles to the treatment of cocaine dependence. *Drug and Alcohol Dependence*, **30**, 87–97.

Hser, Y. I., Grella, C. E., Hubbard, R. L., *et al* (2001) An evaluation of drug treatments for adolescents in four US cities. *Archives of General Psychiatry*, **58**, 689–695.

Hulse, G. K., Robertson, S. I. & Tait, R. J. (2001) Adolescent emergency department presentations with alcohol- or other drug-related problems in Perth, Western Australia. *Addiction*, **96**, 1059–1067.

Joanning, H., Quinn, T. & Mullen, R. (1992) Treating adolescent drug abuse: comparison of family systems therapy, group therapy and family drug education. *Journal of Marital and Family Therapy*, **18**, 345–356.

Kaminer, Y. & Burleson, J. (1999) Psychotherapies for adolescent substance abusers: 15-month follow-up of a pilot study. *American Journal of Addictions*, **8**, 114–119.

——, ——, Blitz, C., *et al* (1998) Psychotherapies for adolescent substance abusers, a pilot study. *Journal of Nervous and Mental Diseases*, **186**, 684–690.

Kazdin, A. (2001) Treatment of conduct disorders. In *Conduct Disorders in Childhood and Adolescence* (eds J. Hill & B. Maughan), pp. 408–448. Cambridge: Cambridge University Press.

King, R. D., Gaines, L. S., Lambert, E. W., *et al* (2000) The co-occurrence of psychiatric and substance use diagnoses in adolescents in different service systems: frequency recognition cost and outcomes. *Journal of Behaviour and Health Services Research*, **27**, 417–430.

Kolvin, I., Garside, R., Nicol, A., *et al* (1981) *Help Starts Here: The Maladjusted Child in the Ordinary School.* London: Tavistock.

Liddle, H., Dakof, G., Parker, K., *et al* (2001) Multidimensional family therapy for adolescent drug abuse: results of a randomized clinical trial. *American Journal of Drug and Alcohol Abuse*, **27**, 651–688.

Longabaugh, R., Woolard, R. F., Nirenberg, T. D. D., *et al* (2001) Evaluating the effects of a brief motivational intervention for injured drinkers in the emergency department. *Journal of Studies on Alcohol*, **63**, 806–816.

McArdle, P., Wiegersma, A., Gilvarry, E., *et al* (2002) Family structure and function and youth drug use. *Addiction*, **97**, 329–336.

McGuire, J. & Priestley, P. (1995) Reviewing 'what works', past, present and future. In *What Works: Reducing Reoffending: Guidelines from Research and Practice* (ed. J. McGuire), pp. 3–34. Chichester: Wiley.

Monti, P. M., Colby, S. M., Barnett, N. P., *et al* (1999) Brief interventions for harm reduction with alcohol positive older adolescents in a hospital emergency department. *Journal of Consulting and Clinical Psychology*, **67**, 989–994.

Myers, M. G., Brown, S. A. & Mott, M. A. (1993) Coping as a predictor of adolescent substance abuse treatment outcome. *Journal of Substance Abuse*, **5**, 15–19.

National Institute for Clinical Excellence (2000) *Guidance on the Use of Methylphenidate (Ritalin, Equasym) for Attention-Deficit/Hyperactivity Disorder in Childhood.* London: National Institute for Clinical Excellence.

—— (2002) *Technology Appraisal Guidance No. 38: Nicotine Replacement Therapy (NRT) and Bupropion for Smoking Cessation.* London: National Institute for Clinical Excellence

O'Brien, C. P. (1997) A range of research based pharmacotherapies for addiction. *Science*, **278**, 66–69.

Piercy, F. P. (1986) *Purdue Brief Family Therapy*. West Lafayette, IN: Center for Institutional Services.

Pliz, J. M. (1992). The development of systems thinking: a historical perspective. In *Systems Perspective*, pp. 45–56. Needham Heights, MA: Allyn & Bacon.

Powell, T., Yeaton, W., Hill, E. M., *et al* (2001) Predictors of psychosocial outcomes for patients with mood disorder: effects of self help group participation. *Psychiatric Rehabilitation*, **25**, 3–11.

Project MATCH Research Group (1997*a*) Matching alcoholism treatments to client heterogeneity: Project MATCH post treatment drinking outcomes. *Journal of Studies on Alcohol*, **58**, 7–29.

—— (1997*b*) Project MATCH secondary a priori hypotheses. *Addiction*, **92**, 1671–1698.

Richmond, R. L. & Anderson, P. (1994) Research in general practice for smokers and excessive drinkers: the experience in Australia and the United Kingdom: 1 Interpreting the results. *Addiction*, **89**, 35–40.

Riggs, P., Mikulich, S., Whitmore, E., *et al* (1999) Relationship of ADHD, depression and non-tobacco substance use disorders to nicotine dependence in substance dependent delinquents. *Drug and Alcohol Dependence*, **54**, 195–205.

Rutter, M. & Rutter, M. (1993) *Developing Minds: Challenges and Continuities Across the Life Span*. New York: Basic Books.

Satterfield, J., Satterfield, B. & Schell, A. M. (1987) Therapeutic interventions to prevent delinquency in hyperactive boys. *Journal of the American Academy of Child and Adolescent Psychiatry*, **26**, 56–64.

Saunders, J. B., Aasland, O. G., Babor, T. F., *et al* (1993) Development of the Alcohol Use Disorders Identification Test (AUDIT): WHO collaborative project on early detection of persons with harmful alcohol consumption: II. *Addiction*, **88**, 791–804.

Schmidt, S. E., Liddle, H. A. & Dakof, G. A. (1996) Changes in parenting practices and adolescent drug abuse during multidimensional family therapy. *Journal of Family Psychology*, **10**, 1–6.

Schoenwald, S. K., Ward, D. M., Henggeler, S. W., *et al* (1996) MST treatment of substance abusing or dependent adolescent offenders: cost of reducing incarceration, inpatient residential placement. *Journal of Child and Family Studies*, **5**, 431–444.

Senft, R. A., Freeborn, D. K., Polen, M. R., *et al* (1997) Brief intervention in a primary care setting for hazardous drinkers. *American Journal of Preventive Medicine*, **13**, 464–470.

Shah, S., Peat, J., Mazurski, E., *et al* (2001) Effect of peer led programmes for asthma education in adolescence, a randomised controlled trial. *British Medical Journal*, **322**, 583–585.

Stanton, M. D. & Shadish, W. R. (1997) Outcome, attrition and family–couples treatment for drug abuse: a meta analysis and review of the controlled, comparative studies. *Psychological Bulletin*, **122**, 170–191.

Stewart, D. G. & Brown, S. (1995) Withdrawal and dependency symptoms among adolescent alcohol and drug abusers. *Addiction*, **90**, 627–635.

Szapocznik, J., Rio, A., Murray, E., *et al* (1989) Structural family versus psychodynamic child therapy for problematic Hispanic boys. *Journal of Consulting and Clinical Psychology*, **57**, 571–578.

Target, M. & Fonagy, P. (1996) The psychological treatment of child and adolescent psychiatric disorders. In *What Works for Whom? A Critical Review of Psychotherapy Research* (eds A. Roth & P. Fonagy), pp. 263–320. New York: Guilford Press.

Wagner, E. F., Brown, S. A., Monti, P. M., *et al* (1999) Innovations in adolescent substance abuse intervention. *Alcoholism: Clinical and Experimental Research*, **23**, 236–249.

Williams, R. & Chang, S. (2000) A comprehensive and comparative review of adolescent substance abuse treatment outcome. *Clinical Psychology: Science and Practice Summary,* **7,** 138–166.

Winters, K. C., Stinchfield, R. D., Opland, E., *et al* (2000) The effectiveness of the Minnesota Model approach in the treatment of adolescent drug abusers. *Addiction,* **95,** 601–612.

Wutzke, S. E., Conigrave, K. M., Saunders, J. B., *et al* (2002) The long term effectiveness of brief interventions for unsafe alcohol consumption: a 10-year follow up. *Addiction,* **97,** 665–675.

CHAPTER 12

Perspectives on substance misuse in young offenders

Sue Bailey and Ruth Marshall

Key points

- Substance misuse is an identified risk factor for the development of offending behaviour.
- Associations are recognised between substance misuse and various forms of psychopathology.
- High levels of substance misuse are seen in populations of young sex offenders.
- Young people with antisocial behaviour need a thorough mental health needs assessment, including assessment of their substance misuse.
- To enable services to respond equitably to the complex, unmet needs of young offenders, including their substance misuse, there will have to be considerable investment, particularly in training.

Background

Young people who are arrested for delinquent behaviour may or may not meet diagnostic criteria for a conduct disorder or oppositional defiant disorder. Both require a pattern of multiple antisocial behaviours over an extended period of time. Equally, young people diagnosed with conduct or oppositional defiant disorder may or may not have any contact with the juvenile justice system or be designated as delinquents *per se*. Nevertheless, the reality is that there is often considerable overlap in the antisocial behaviours of both delinquent and conduct-disordered young people. There is also considerable variation in how young people start on one particular pathway of interventions, successful or otherwise, in the jurisdictions of education, health, social care and juvenile justice. In reality, a specific behaviour is identified as problematic because of its consequences for others or the young person, and it is this and other possible behaviours that lead to a response, or lack of response in some cases, from either the mental health or the juvenile justice system.

More than one developmental path can lead to clinically severe antisocial behaviour in young people. In his seminal paper, Loeber (1990) delineated three distinct pathways:

- the *aggressive–versatile path*, which begins in the pre-school years and involves a great variety of aggressive and non-aggressive conduct problems, as well as hyperactivity (this pathway has been labelled by other authors as 'early starter' (Patterson *et al*, 1991), 'life-course persistent' (Moffitt, 1993) and 'childhood onset' (Hinshaw *et al*, 1993));
- the *non-aggressive path*, which begins in late childhood or early adolescence, and primarily involves non-aggressive conduct problems (theft, lying, truancy, substance misuse) that are often committed in the company of deviant peers;

Table 12.1 Factors linked with antisocial behaviour

Individual characteristics	Family characteristics	Peer relations	School factors	Neighbourhood and community characteristics
Poor verbal skills	Lack of monitoring	Association with deviant peers	Low achievement	High mobility
Favourable attitude towards antisocial behaviour	Ineffective discipline	Poor relationship skills	Drop-out from school	Little support available from neighbours and community organisations
Psychiatric symptoms	Low warmth	Low association with pro-social peers	Low commitment to education	High disorganisation
Cognitive bias to attribute hostile intentions to others	High conflict		Weak structure and chaotic environments	Criminal subculture
	Parental difficulties – drug misuse, psychiatric morbidity, criminality			

Source: adapted with permission from the work of Scott Henggeler and colleagues.

- the *exclusive substance misuse path*, which begins in early to middle adolescence and involves no appreciable antecedent conduct problems.

With ongoing research, refinement of these different developmental pathways will no doubt proceed (Bronfenbrenner, 1979). However, the above gives a basic framework for the core issues that affect those young people who are offending and misusing substances.

Empirical research (Rutter *et al*, 1998) demonstrates that serious antisocial behaviour is determined by the reciprocal interaction of characteristics of the individual young person and the key social systems in which the young person's life is played out. The factors linked with antisocial behaviour are relatively constant (Table 12.1), whether the behaviour examined is conduct disorder, delinquency or substance misuse (Hawkins *et al*, 1992; Bailey, 2003; Farrington, 2003.

Findings from both the field of delinquency and that of substance misuse (Henggeler *et al*, 1998) show that aggression and other conduct problems in early adolescence foreshadow adult criminal behaviour.

Long-term social and economic costs of antisocial behaviour

Kratzer & Hodgkins (1997) found that conduct problems during early adolescence predicted both criminality and mental disorders, mainly substance misuse, at the age of 30 years. Although the economic costs of adult antisocial behaviour are difficult to estimate, they are undoubtedly substantial and can be seen in the funding involved in the following areas:

- the cost of housing an adult prison population;
- the cost of law enforcement;
- the cost of victimisation from serious antisocial behaviour, which involves not only physical injury to victims of violent crime but also the psychological damage and lost productivity within the workforce.

Young people who engage in antisocial delinquent behaviours are at increased risk of several deleterious outcomes during adulthood, including substance misuse and dependence.

Policy and law in England and Wales

That growing numbers of young people are becoming involved in crime has been known for many years and across many countries. As a result, new policies are continually being introduced in the youth justice field.

There has been ongoing debate about the efficacy of custody and preventive community programmes, and increasingly governments have sought ways to make parents responsible for the criminal behaviour of their children. For example, the Youth Justice Board (YJB) was established in England and Wales following implementation of the Crime and Disorder Act 1998 (Ashford & Chard, 2000) and has been given statutory responsibility to set standards and to advise the Home Secretary on all matters relating to the youth justice system. This includes:

- wide-ranging powers to oversee youth justice initiatives;
- responsibility to improve the way offending behaviour is dealt with;
- finding ways to reduce offending;
- streamlining court procedures;
- introducing and monitoring the new multi-disciplinary teams (youth offending teams, or YOTS) which deal with young offenders in the community;
- improving the standard of secure provision for juveniles given a custodial sentence by the courts.

The YJB commissions and purchases secure accommodation for all those under 18 years old sentenced or remanded by the courts. Between April 2000 and April 2001, there was a 7% increase in the number of people under 18 years of age held in custody. The unexpectedly high use of the detention training orders introduced in April 2000 has meant that the YJB was unable to meet its commitment to remove all young girls from prison by April 2001, although a long-term commitment to do so was restated. There are, on average, 11 000 young people (defined as under 21 years of age) held in prison at any one time, of whom 500 are female and nearly 3000 are children, as defined by the Children Act 1989 (the Act defines a child as any person under the age of 18). Young Black people are overrepresented in both the prison and mental health systems. Home Office statistics on race show that around 20% of prisoners under 21 years of age are from Black and minority ethnic groups (Home Office, 1999).

When dealing with young people within the juvenile justice system, the relevant legislative frameworks are as follows: the Children Act 1989 states that the welfare of the child is paramount and should be safeguarded and promoted; area child protection committees (ACPCs), which emphasise the importance of close liaison between the prison service and social services departments in the assessment of children in need and their families; and the Human Rights Act 1998, as well as international law, including the United Nations Convention on the Rights of the Child, which was ratified by the UK government as far back as 1991, which set out the rights of children.

The age of criminal responsibility in England and Wales is 10 years; in Scotland it is currently under review. The ages of criminal responsibility are significantly lower in the UK than in many other countries. Section 34 of the Crime and Disorder Act 1998 abolished the refutable presumption that a child is *doli incapa*: that is, incapable of telling the difference between serious wrong and simple naughtiness. For the purposes of the criminal law this means that children over the age of criminal responsibility are seen as being as responsible as their adult counterparts.

Multiple needs

We know that young people in custody are in poor mental health compared with those in the general population. Over 50% of young men on remand and 30% of sentenced young men have a diagnosable mental disorder (HM Chief Inspector of Prisons, 1997). Imprisonment itself has been identified as having a negative impact on the mental health of young offenders (Mental Health Foundation, 1999). The Office of National Statistics' survey of psychiatric morbidity among young offenders (aged 16–20 years) in England and Wales (Lader et al, 2000) found high levels of psychiatric disorder (Table 12.2).

Failing to meet the mental health needs of young people in the community, including those with substance misuse problems, can lead to them becoming embroiled in the criminal justice system and all too often ending up in the prison system. Street (2000) highlighted the problems of meeting the mental health needs of young people in the community:

* referral rates to mental health services were greatly increased, including the numbers of emergencies;
* there was increased pressure on all community services, especially consultant child and adolescent psychiatrists;

Table 12.2 Psychiatric morbidity among young offenders

	Prevalence among prisoners	
	on remand (%)	convicted (%)
Any personality disorder (DSM–IV SCID-II)	84	88
Psychotic and severe affective disorder (SCAN)	8	10
Neurotic disorders (CIS-R): sleep problems, worry (not about physical health), irritability, depression	52	41

Source: Lader et al (2000). Crown copyright; reproduced with permission.

- confusion and frustration were experienced by those dealing with children who have conduct disorders and challenging behaviour, including substance misuse.

The combination of youth, mental health problems, substance misuse and offending attracts a great deal of media and parliamentary attention and concern. Many children and young people arrive in secure accommodation with a complex history of disturbance and distress. There is frequently a web of risk factors in these young people's lives, and their mental health problems need to be seen in the context of a range of other problems.

Understanding the young person in the context of life experiences will help in meeting needs and may in turn have a positive effect on their mental health (see Chapter 11). By understanding and addressing the range of difficulties these young people face, including social disadvantage, one needs to understand the overlap between risk factors for mental ill health, offending behaviour and substance misuse. This has been most clearly identified in the Audit Commission's (1996) report *Mis-spent Youth*. The risk factors for offending were made explicit:

- inadequate parental supervision;
- problems in school, such as truancy or exclusion;
- mixing with others who offend;
- lack of a stable family home;
- aggressive hyperactive behaviour;
- lack of employment or education;
- misuse of alcohol or drugs.

This is in keeping with the vast research in the area. We know that problems with substance misuse are highest among young offenders who are sentenced (Lader *et al*, 2000). The 1998 British Crime Survey (Ramsey & Partridge, 1999) found that in the 16–19-year age group, 55% of males and 42% of females had tried an illicit drug, whereas in the incarcerated population, 96% of sentenced young men and 84% of sentenced young women had tried illicit drugs. The distinct message from all of this work being done on young offenders in custody and in the community is that mental health and substance misuse services should not operate in ways that exclude young people in need of their help. The issues remain pragmatics, lack of resources, lack of workforce skills and lack of a strategic mechanism to ensure that appropriate professionals can be recruited, trained and retained to deliver fit-for-purpose services in this challenging field.

The YJB has developed an assessment tool, ASSET (Youth Justice Board, 2000), for use by youth offending teams and all those working within the juvenile secure estate. Emotional and mental health needs are covered, as is substance misuse, but the YJB recognises the need to develop a more specific mental health screening and surveillance tool that can encompass substance misuse screens. This work is now being undertaken by the Research and Clinical Adolescent Forensic Team based at the University of Manchester (Kroll *et al*, 2002). Youth offending teams are expected to use ASSET to assess all young people with whom they are working. This assessment accompanies young offenders as they move in and between systems within the criminal justice system. Although a number of criticisms have been levelled at ASSET, mainly based on difficulties in completion, it is an important step forward in providing a baseline understanding of the risks and needs of young children entering the criminal justice system.

Under the Crime and Disorder Act 1998, health authorities must contribute to the operation of youth offending teams. However, their contribution has been variable. Some youth offending teams have a health visitor to look at early interventions, general health and support to families. Others have a clinical nurse specialist working with older adolescents around particular mental health problems, including substance misuse, or experienced substance misuse counsellors working as part of the youth offending team. However, even when problems have been identified, this does not answer the question of resources and what services these young people they can move on to. Certainly, a better assessment of mental health and substance misuse problems has to be developed. The tool being developed by the Manchester team will be based on the needs of the young person and not simply on diagnosis.

Thus, mental health assessment should ascertain whether any substance, or range of substances, including prescribed medication and alcohol, are being misused. Use of substances must not exclude someone from mental health services. Such assessment will require adequate guidelines and training, which will need to be provided within the criminal justice system as a whole.

Substance misuse and antisocial behaviour

Many studies have demonstrated associations between adolescent drug and alcohol use and various forms of psychopathology, including low self-esteem, depression, antisocial behaviour, aggressiveness, crime and poor school performance (Angold *et al*, 1999). Indeed, many studies of antisocial behaviour still include early drug use as one of a range of possible symptoms. Young people who later become problem drinkers have often been found to have high rates of school drop-out and poor achievement.

Substance misuse and antisocial behaviour increase in frequency over the same adolescent age period, and the two have also shown a parallel rise over the past 50 years (Rutter & Smith, 1995). To a considerable extent, they also involve similar risk factors, and it seems reasonable therefore to regard them both as part of the same underlying propensity to engage in socially disapproved behaviour (Jessor & Jessor, 1977). Studies of temporal ordering have found that the onset of antisocial behaviour generally precedes alcohol or substance misuse, and Gittelman *et al* (1985) and Loeber (1990) concluded that twice as many delinquents initiated drug use after their delinquent involvement compared with those initiating delinquency after drug use. In other words, antisocial behaviour seems to predispose to illicit drug taking.

But does the converse also apply? Does taking drugs increase the likelihood of criminality? There is evidence that it does, both because of peer group pressure and because stealing may be necessary to finance the purchase of certain kinds of drugs. The complexity of this association is illustrated from Cohen and Brooks' (1987) longitudinal study of primary schoolchildren in New York. They found that childhood aggression was associated with an increased risk of later substance misuse, and substance misuse in adolescence increased the risk of subsequent delinquency, even when childhood aggression was taken into account. On the basis of these data, the authors concluded that, in addition to shared risk factors, drug use predisposed to crime through several mechanisms. First, it helped reduce inhibitions. Secondly, it created a need for money to purchase drugs. Thirdly, it created a peer group culture that fostered further drug use and delinquency. It seems, then, that both alcohol and drug misuse show a substantial association with crime, with bidirectional course and processes.

Antisocial behaviour is commonly associated with other kinds of mental health problems, particularly attention-deficit hyperactivity disorder, affective disorders and substance misuse. In planning mental health services for juvenile offenders, therefore, it is necessary not only to consider interventions that reduce offending, but also to consider treatments for non-antisocial behaviours. In this context, it is important to recognise that there should be no assumption that treatment of non-antisocial behaviours will necessarily reduce the risk of offending. Although we know relatively little of the mechanisms linking antisocial behaviour and problems such as emotional disorders and substance misuse, it is probable that at least part of the association stems from shared risk factors, such as family background and neighbourhood influences. In other cases, such as depression, it is likely that the comorbid disorder is in some sense secondary to antisocial behaviour. Treatment of these comorbid problems will not necessarily therefore reduce offending.

Nevertheless, there are other instances, most notably attention-deficit hyperactivity disorder, where, at least in theory, it is reasonable to suppose that effective treatment of a comorbid disorder may lower the risks of later antisocial behaviour.

Multi-systemic therapy for young people with serious antisocial behaviour

A framework is presented here for how services could and should be delivered to those young people entering the criminal justice system who also have significant substance misuse problems. The framework has largely been constructed on the basis of the following reviews of recent research, experience and initiatives: Farrant (2001) and Standing Conference on Drug Abuse (1999a,b, 2000). The framework centres on the application of multi-systemic therapy (MST) to young people with serious antisocial behaviour (Henggeler et al, 1998; Borduin, 1999).

Many of the young people who are referred for MST have serious antisocial behaviour: they engage in impulsive and aggressive acts. Usually these behaviours diminish in both frequency and intensity when both ecological and systemic interventions are implemented. In some cases, however, impulsive or aggressive behaviours continue even after changes in the youth's social ecology. In such cases the practitioner and family need to take stock of the multi-systemic interventions in place to ensure that they are targeting all factors contributing to the 'fit' of impulsive or aggressive behaviour, and that the interventions are being implemented consistently by all the key players – not just the parents but also those involved from other jurisdictions. If problem behaviour continues to surface, then an enhanced programme needs to be developed that deals more directly with the individual characteristics of the adolescent. Individual therapy with the adolescent can be carried out but still using the general overarching MST principle of assessing the fit of social cognition with problem behaviours.

Research on aggressive and impulsive youths indicates that they experience some distortions and deficiencies in social cognition that contribute to their aggression. For example, they pay more attention to aggressive cues in the environment, and attribute the behaviour of others to hostile intentions even when that behaviour is neutral (this constitutes the distortion). They come up with fewer verbally assertive (this is a deficit) and more physically aggressive solutions to social problems. They are more likely to label arousal as anger rather than fear or sadness (Kendall, 1993). Whether youth justice workers are centred in youth offending teams, local authority secure units or youth offender institutions, it is commonplace now to hear workers discuss the use of 'anger management'. Practitioners will try to work with the young person in an effort to manage anger, 'teach him to walk away' or 'count to ten'. From an MST perspective and from what is known about social cognitive processes, such goals and interventions plans are likely to fail because:

- they do not address the sequence of interactions that led to the angry or aggressive outbursts;
- they overlook the role of cognitive distortions and the sequence of events punctuated by physical or verbal aggression.

Within the framework of MST, targeting family interactions and cognitive distortions can provide opportunities to prevent angry or aggressive outbursts. This is better than relying solely on helping the youth and family members to manage the anger and threatening behaviour after it has occurred. Cognitive–behavioural interventions which involve the MST principles can enable the practitioner and the young person to collaborate in thinking through, and to practise, solutions to the specific interpersonal problems targeted for change. The main objective of individual sessions is to identify and address those distortions and deficiencies that compromise the young person's ability to develop, choose and implement solutions to internal problems, that is, the distortions and deficiencies that result in negative outcomes for the young person and others, even when ecological interventions to help the family deal with difficulties are already in place. Cognitive–behavioural interventions to accomplish these aims generally draw on five classes of strategies, as described in Kendall's (1993) work:

- modelling
- role-play exercise
- behavioural contingencies
- self-monitoring and self-instruction
- problem-solving training – which combines all these strategies to teach individuals to engage in a sequential and deliberate process of solving problems that arise in social interactions.

The therapist can implement these strategies in the context of individual sessions but can also actively engage parents and teachers in anticipating and reinforcing (using behavioural contingencies and verbal praise). The change is initiated in individual meetings with the young person. To this end, the therapist describes to the parent the specific skills being modelled, taught and practised in individual sessions, and asks the parent to watch for and concretely reinforce instances during the day in which the young person has tried to use the skill (Henggler *et al*, 1997).

Problem-solving training

When aggressive or impulsive behaviour is associated with a failure to think (or at least to think enough) before acting, problem-solving training can help adolescents think for themselves and act in a non-impulsive manner. The essential steps of most problem-solving approaches are:

- Identify the problem, including all relevant emotional (feelings in a situation), social (who is present, in what social context), and environmental aspects of the problem situation.
- Determine the young person's goals in the problem situation.
- Generate alternative solutions.
- Evaluate these solutions.
- Choose, practise and implement a plan for the solution.
- Evaluate the plan, and redesign as needed.

However, before using these strategies the therapist must assess the young person's level of cognitive development. With younger children and adolescents with low levels of cognitive ability, a behavioural approach that teaches the child how to use the steps is to be preferred to an extensive analysis of how the problem-solving process itself works. With more mature children and more able adolescents, the therapist can facilitate generalisation of skills by including more work on the reasons why the problem-solving process can be effective.

Identify the problem

The main objectives of this first step are to describe:

- the problem in terms of real situations that occur in the young person's life;
- the situational details of what happens over time in the situation;
- the thoughts, feelings and behaviours the youth experiences as the situation unfolds;
- the characteristics of the situation that make it a problem.

In an MST model, the therapist would already have ample observations and reports from others of real situations in the youth's life that can serve to exemplify the problem. Using these exemplars. the therapist and the young person can describe the problem in terms of antecedents, behaviours of concern and consequences – immediate, medium term and long term. The therapist helps the adolescent to identify the interrelationship between thoughts, feelings and behaviours as they arise over time in the problem situation, so that the young person can be more aware of his or her own impact on problem situations. The therapist can also help the young person identify what makes this problem a problem, that is, the negative consequences experienced either by others or by the young person.

Determine the goals

The therapist has to focus on goals – given a specific problem, what is the outcome to be achieved? The criteria, which must be discussed fully with the young person, are that goals should be assertive, reflect the feelings or opinions of the young person, and avoid both aggression and passivity. It is generally best to consider both improving something as well as decreasing something.

Generate alternative solutions

This step consists of brainstorming. The goal is to have the young person, with or without assistance, generate a list that includes solutions that might actually work and options that would probably lead to negative consequences. It is important to have criteria for the brainstorming:

- No idea is evaluated until the list is complete.
- The list should include realistic, unrealistic and even non-options.
- Aggressive, assertive and passive options are required.

The therapist should emphasise having fun and encourage the young person to ask others, especially those who are socially desirable, for help in generating options.

Evaluate the solutions

Once the list is developed the therapist asks the young person to evaluate each option. Only assertive options can be considered acceptable. The young person is instructed to cross out any aggressive, inappropriate options. Passive options may be acceptable, particularly in situations that involve confrontation with those in authority. The possible consequences of each option (again, immediate, medium and long term), for others as well as the young person, are then listed and discussed, and their relative merits evaluated.

Choose, practise and implement a plan

The therapist reviews the relative strengths and weaknesses of the solutions with the young person and helps to design a plan. All positive options should be considered. Either one or a combination of positive options can be used for the plan, which should be described in behaviourally specific terms of who does what, when and where. Developing and practising sample scripts is helpful when talking with another person. Role-play, practice, praise and constructive feedback are required if the implementation of the plan is to have any chance of succeeding.

The therapist helps the young person to implement the plan by a particular date and all details are discussed. In some instances, the therapist can go with the young person and provide support, although in the long run the young person needs to learn this set of skills in order to accomplish all the steps on his or her own.

Evaluate the plan

Therapists have to enlist support from significant carers in encouraging the youth and in checking to see whether she/he has been able to execute the plan in real life. If at first it does not work, the therapist helps the young person to re-evaluate and redesign the plan. Such reconceptualisations require the youth to develop the skills to evaluate his or her performance objectively. This can be the most difficult stage for the young person who is less able and less motivated to accept help. The therapist here has to model and encourage the use of self-monitoring statements that are specific and objective, such as 'I didn't use assertive statements' rather than 'I just made a mess of it'. If the plan is successful, the therapist encourages the youth to describe the basis for the success and emphasises internal attribution for the outcome.

Addressing cognitive distortions

With aggressive and impulsive youths, particularly those who have moved on into significant substance misuse, addressing cognitive distortions is the most difficult aspect of intervention. The range of interventions in this arena is now legion. The most difficult step is defining the starting point. It may be useful to start by trying to understand how this particular young person 'takes in' a social situation:

*   Does the young person tune into hostile or negative cues in the environment much of the time?
*   Does the young person interpret behaviours that may be neutral or mildly negative as being motivated by hostile intentions? For example, is a sidelong glance perceived as an invitation to fight?

This information can be best obtained by accompanying the young person to a variety of social settings (playing sport, eating out, in a shopping centre) that afford opportunities to watch him or her interact. The therapist could then ask, for example, 'Why do you think that that person over there is acting in that particular way?' The need is to gain from the young person an idea of how he or she thinks the other person whose behaviour is being observed is feeling, and ask the young person what he or she thinks that person will do next.'

When distortions such as hostile attributions generalise across different types of people and situations they can become attitudinal biases. For instance, some juvenile offenders may believe their teachers and the police are 'out to get them'. The tone of voice and other subtle or overtly hostile behaviour they exhibit on the basis of the distorted cognition and the feelings of anger, persecution or hostility associated with this attribution in turn often evoke hostility from peers and adults alike. This hostility serves to reinforce the adolescent's belief. This is particularly heightened where the young person is taking substances, especially if this is getting them in trouble with the law, or is beginning to generate feelings of paranoia.

In such circumstances, the adolescent has to learn that his or her body posture, tone of voice and behaviours contribute to this cycle of hostile interactions. To provoke this understanding the therapist can use a variety of perspective-taking exercises, including Socratic methods, that enhance the young person's appreciation of the other person's perspective. The therapist is therefore attempting to teach the adolescent that in many situations his or her negative attitude and behaviour force adult authorities to respond in the appointed fashion. Adolescents who are able to understand the connection between their behaviour and the responses of others are then capable of learning, even if only at a basic level, 'how to play the game'.

This type of approach has value for the majority of juvenile offenders who are also misusing substances. Care has to be taken, however, with that small group of young people whose conduct disorder is characterised by cold, unemotional responses to those around them, those who, with a combination of substance misuse, are at risk not of an adult antisocial personality disorder but of an adult psychopathic personality disorder. For that small group, learning to play the game may not be the desired outcome, as they will not use this to positive but to negative ends. This reinforces the need for very careful individual assessment of every young offender by people with expertise in a developmental approach to child and adolescent mental health.

Conclusions

Our understanding of developmental pathways into antisocial behaviour is developing rapidly. The factors linked with antisocial behaviour are relatively constant, whether the behaviour being described is conduct disorder, delinquency or substance misuse. Tackling such behaviour is of paramount importance for the future adult health and well-being of today's antisocial youths and the health of their victims; it also has the potential to avoid enormous social and economic costs to both society and subsequent generations.

Failed, fragmented responses of the education, health and social services have led to large numbers of young people entering the criminal justice system, bringing with them their mental health problems, destructive substance misuse and complex unmet needs. The challenge set by recent government initiatives in the health and criminal justice systems will place considerable demands on health practitioners working in the fields of both child and adolescent mental health services and addiction psychiatry.

The extent and meaning of the association between offending and substance misuse, although apparent, remains complex, multi-layered, and difficult to disentangle when it comes to practical interventions.

When combined, serious antisocial behaviour and substance misuse are likely both to lead a young person into conflict with the law and to jeopardise health. Any systematic attempt to intervene successfully with this group will be characterised by the following:

- The process of careful mental health needs assessment is repeated over time and through contexts.
- Mental health education, which covers substance misuse, is disseminated to non-mental health practitioners.
- Training and education are delivered in a manner that enables multi-agency practitioners to be alert to, and more confident in the assessment of, young people at risk who require referral to more specialist services.
- The overall aim should be to enable health practitioners to respond to unmet needs in a way that allows equity of access to services whatever the background and geographical location of the young person. For this to happen, resources and expertise have to be effectively channelled into developing a skilled, fit-for-purpose mental health workforce. Bringing together the skills of additional psychiatry and child and adolescent mental health services is an essential first step in this process.
- The intervention has to based on an understanding of adolescents in a developmental context and an appreciation of the impact of the not uncommon findings of hostile attributions of many young offenders, derived from the chaos and abuse which has character-ised their childhood lives.

Acknowledgements

The first author acknowledges with thanks the work of Scott Henggeler and colleagues (treatment manuals for practitioners) and the training undertaken as a multi-systemic therapist in South Carolina in 2000.

References

Angold, A., Costello, E. J. & Erkanli, A. (1999) Comorbidity. *Journal of Child Psychology and Psychiatry*, **40**, 57–87.

Ashford, M. & Chard, A. (2000) *Defending Young People in the Criminal Justice System* (2nd edn). London: Legal Action Group.

Audit Commission (1996) *Mis-spent Youth*. London: Audit Commission.

Bailey (2003) Young offenders and mental health. *Current Opinion in Psychiatry*, **16**, 581–591.

Borduin, C. M. (1999) Multisystemic treatment of criminality and violence in adolescents. *Journal of the American Academy for Child and Adolescent Psychiatry*, **50**, 242–249.

Bronfenbrenner, U. (1979) *The Ecology of Human Development*. Cambridge, MA: Harvard University Press.

Cohen, P. & Brooks, S. (1987) Family factors related to the persistence of psycho-pathology in childhood and adolescence. *Psychiatry*, **50**, 332–345.

Farrant, F. (2001) *Troubled Inside: Responding to the Mental Health Needs of Children and Young People in Prison*. London: Prison Reform Trust.

Farrington, D. P. (2002) Key results from the first forty years of the Cambridge study of delinquent development. In *Taking Stock of Delinquency: An Overview* (eds T. P. Thornberry & M. D. Krohn), pp. 137–183. New York: Kluwer Plenum Academic Publishers.

—— (2003) Advancing knowledge about the early prevention of adult antisocial behaviour. In *Early Prevention of Adult Antisocial Behaviour* (eds D. P. Farrington & J. W. Coid). Cambridge: Cambridge University Press.

Gittelman, R., Mannuzza, S., Shenker, R., *et al* (1985) Hyperactive boys almost grown up I: Psychiatric status. *Archives of General Psychiatry*, **42**, 937–947.

Hawkins, J. D., Catalano, R. F. & Miller, J. Y. (1992) Risk and protective factors for alcohol and other drugs problems in adolescence and early adulthood: implications for substance abuse prevention. *Physiological Bulletin*, **112**, 64–105.

Henggeler, S. W., Melton, G. B., Brondino, M. J., *et al* (1997) Multi systemic therapy with violent and chronic juvenile offenders and their families: the role of treatment fidelity in successful dissemination. *Journal of Consulting and Clinical Physiology*, **65**, 821–833.

——, Schoenwald, S. K., Borduin, C. M., *et al* (1998) *Multi-systemic Treatment of Antisocial Behaviour in Children and Adolescents*. London: Guilford Press.

Hinshaw, S. P., Lehey, B. B. & Hart, E. L. (1993) Issues of taxonomy and co-morbidity in the development of conduct disorder. *Development and Psychopathology*, **5**, 31–49.

HM Chief Inspector of Prisons (1997) *Young Prisoners: A Thematic Review*. London: Home Office.

Home Office (1999) *Statistics on Race in the Criminal Justice System*. London: The Stationery Office.

Jessor, R. & Jessor, S. (1977) *Problem Behavior and Psychosocial Development: A Longitudinal Study of Youth*. New York: Academic Press.

Kendall, P. C. (1993) Cognitive–behavioural therapies with youth: guiding theory, current status and emerging developments. *Journal of Consulting and Clinical Psychology*, **61**, 235–247.

Kratzer, L. & Hodgkins, S. (1997) Adult outcomes of child conduct problems: a cohort study. *Journal of Abnormal Child Psychology*, **25**, 65–81.

Kroll, L., Rothwell, J., Bradley, D., *et al* (2002) Mental health needs of boys in secure care for serious or persistent offending: a prospective, longitudinal study. *Lancet*, **359**, 1978–1979.

Lader, D., Singleton, N. & Meltzer, H. (2000) *Psychiatric Morbidity Among Young Offenders in England and Wales: Further Analysis of Data from the ONS Survey of Psychiatric Morbidity Among Prisoners in England and Wales Carried Out in 1997 on Behalf of the Department of Health*. London: Office for National Statistics.

Loeber, R. (1990) Development and risk factors of juvenile antisocial behaviour and delinquency. *Clinical Psychology Review*, **10**, 1–41.

Mental Health Foundation (1999) *Bright Futures: Promoting Young People's Mental Health*. London: Saltzberg–Wittenberg.

Moffitt, T. E. (1993) Adolescence-limited and life-course-persistent antisocial behaviour: a developmental taxonomy. *Psychological Review*, **100**, 674–701.

Patterson, G. R., Kapaldi, D. & Bank, L. (1991) An early starter model for predicting delinquency. In *The Development and Treatment of Childhood Aggression* (eds D. J. Peppler & K .H. Rubin), pp. 139–168. Hillsdale, NJ: Earlbaum.

Ramsey, M. & Partridge, S. (1999) *Drug Misuse Declared in 1998: Results from the British Crime Survey*. London: Home Office.

Rutter, M. & Smith, D. (1995) *Psychosocial Disorders in Young People: Time Trends and Their Causes*. Chichester: Wiley.

——, Giller, H. & Hagell, A. (1998) Antisocial behaviour by young people. *Varieties of Antisocial Behaviour*, **5**, 95–126.

Standing Conference on Drug Abuse (1999a) *Drugs and Young Offenders: Guidance for Drug Action Teams and Youth Offender Teams*. London: Home Office, Drugs Prevention Advisory Service.

—— (1999b) *Young People and Drugs: Policy Guidance in Drug Interventions*. London: Standing Conference on Drug Abuse, Children's Legal Centre.

—— (2000) *Assessing Young People's Drug Taking: Guidance for Drug Services*. London: Standing Conference on Drug Abuse.

Street, C. (2000) *Whose Crisis?* London: Young Minds.

Youth Justice Board (2000) *ASSET*. London: Youth Justice Board.

CHAPTER 13

Ethical and legal principles

Carole A. Kaplan and Paul McArdle

Key points

- There is a complex legislative framework within which all professionals work in the area of substance misuse by young people, which is different to that applied to adults. Guidelines are also in existence and these must be noted.
- All professionals have a duty to know the framework within which they work and deviations from these require justification.
- Consent to treatment should be judged on capacity, not age alone. In rare cases, the courts may override refusal to accept treatment.
- In dealing with confidentiality, the interests of the child must be considered alongside his or her rights.
- All services must be accountable for their work with children and young people. Working in professional isolation and using unusual approaches should be avoided, and if there is significant variation from their usual practice this must be checked and explained.

Introduction

The current legal framework in England and Wales can be perceived as both a help and a hindrance to professionals working in the field of substance misuse and child health. There is a distinctive framework within which we all are bound, but the age-old consideration that that which is legal is not necessarily ethical must enter this debate.

This chapter addresses the legislative framework in terms of the Acts concerning the use of alcohol and drugs and the Mental Health Act, including some potential consequences of the proposals for a new Act. However, the principles of the Children Act remain at the heart of legal provision for the welfare of children. The assessment of risk of harm is considered, as are issues relating to consent and competence to give consent, and the problems of confidentiality. The key principles for professional assessment and intervention are outlined and finally the implications for the structure of services are reviewed.

All professionals and individual citizens have obligations and responsibilities under the law. Disagreement with the law does not confer the right to act unlawfully. With regard to patients and clients, the principle that the law has been formulated in the best interests of society must be respected, even if not always agreed with. It should also be noted that children and adolescents have the right to expect that we will practise within the law.

Guidelines formulated or adopted by a variety of authoritative bodies do not have the force of law. Nevertheless, to behave in breach of these may have consequences. There is increasing pressure to account for the way that we practise. This includes the need to demonstrate that not only is this of an acceptable standard but also that it is open to scrutiny and, if necessary, to modification.

There is also a wider professional, and even personal, imperative to try to shape society in a better way for young people and their future. This may have a goal of modification of laws and guidelines. Furthermore, we have a privilege of advocacy for those we see professionally, particularly when they are children and adolescents.

The legislative framework

The Children Act 1989 is aimed directly at those caring for and protecting children. Other Acts, such as the Human Rights Act 1998, the Misuse of Drugs Act 1971, the Family Law Act 1996 and the Race Relations Act 1976, with their amendments, may also affect children and the way adults respond to them.

The Youth Justice and Criminal Evidence Act 1999 provides for referral orders, the establishment of youth offender panels and specialist court proceedings, and describes the function of youth offender teams. A referral order applies where a youth court or other magistrates' court is dealing with a person under the age of 18 years for an offence for which neither a custodial sentence nor absolute discharge is being proposed. The contract may include provision for unpaid work in the community, attendance at school or other establishment, and participation in specified activities, such as rehabilitation programmes for those dependent on or having a propensity to misuse alcohol or drugs. Any such programme must involve both child practitioners and those with skills in drug misuse and addiction. It is important that they represent partnerships between local young people's services and drug and alcohol services (Gilvarry *et al*, 2001). A further section encompasses a power to restrict reporting of criminal proceedings involving persons under 18.

The Criminal Justice and Police Act 2001 includes provisions for combating alcohol-related disorder. These include the use of alcohol in designated public places. They refer to the closure of licensed premises, the confiscation of alcohol containers from young people, the sale of intoxicating liquor to those under 18, and the enforcement of certain penalties, for example with regard to drunkenness on licensed premises. The use of alcohol in public areas, particularly parks, is frequently observed among young people who drink outside of parental control. (The Confiscation of Alcohol (Young Persons) Act 1997 also provides the police with a power of confiscation where young people are drinking in public.)

The Act 2001 makes amendments to the Licensing Act 1964, with regard to sale of alcohol to young people under 18 years. Under the Licensing Act 1964, it is an offence to sell or supply alcohol to persons under the age of 18 years in licensed premises, and an offence for the minor to purchase or attempt to purchase alcoholic beverages. This has actually been the law since the Intoxicating Liquor Act 1923. Despite this legislation, children continue to obtain alcohol with ease. A voluntary introduction of 'proof of age' has been welcomed but is too often ignored (80% of surveys have shown that, even with proof of age, minors have still been able to purchase alcohol). The 2001 Act further provides for combating crime such as drug trafficking, use of controlled drugs in certain premises and advertisements relating to prostitution. It is hoped that enforcement of such legislation will protect young people, reduce youth crime associated with alcohol, improve public protection and support national targets with regard to health, education and employment for young people.

The Licensing (Young Persons) Act 2000 also states that any person who sells or knowingly allows the sale of alcohol to a person under 18 commits an offence. The adult is now expected to prove that he or she believed the person was not under age, or took reasonable steps to establish the person's age, or that nobody could reasonably expect from the young person's appearance that he or she was under 18. It is now also an offence to buy or attempt to buy alcohol in licensed premises on behalf of a person under 18.

An intoxicated young person may be arrested and a medical practitioner asked to judge that person's fitness for interview. A joint report of the Association of Police Surgeons & Royal College of Psychiatrists (2000) proposed certain guidelines on this. A detainee may be unfit for interview when conducting an interview could worsen any existing physical or mental illness to a significant degree. Alternatively, anything said or done by the detainee at the time of detention may be considered unreliable in subsequent court proceedings because of the physical or mental state of the detainee. The report indicates that this may be because of intoxication or withdrawal and the risk of, for instance, a false confession.

Table 13.1 Summary of the classes of drugs set out in the Misuse of Drugs Act 1971

Class	Main drugs in class	Maximum penalties for possession	Maximum penalties for possession with intent to supply
A	Heroin, cocaine (and crack cocaine), ecstasy, LSD, methadone, morphine, opium, dipipanone, pethidine, cannabinol, and cannabinol derivatives, Class B drugs when designed for injection	In a magistrates' court: six-month prison sentence, a fine of £5000, or both In a trial by jury: seven-year prison sentence, an unlimited fine, or both	In a magistrates' court: six-month prison sentence, a fine of £5000, or both In a trial by jury: Life sentence, an unlimited fine, or both
B	Amphetamines, barbiturates, cannabis[1] (herbal and resin), codeine, dihydrocodeine and methylamphetamine	In a magistrates' court: three-month prison sentence, a fine of £2500, or both In a trial by jury: five-year sentence, an unlimited fine, or both	In a magistrates' court: six-month prison sentence, a fine of £5000, or both In a trial by jury: 14-year sentence, an unlimited fine, or both
C	Benzodiazepines, buprenorphine, diethylpropion, anabolic steroids	In a magistrates' court: three-month prison sentence, a fine of £1000, or both In a trial by jury: two-year sentence, an unlimited fine, or both	In a magistrates' court: three-month prison sentence, a fine of £2500, or both In a trial by jury: five-year sentence, an unlimited fine, or both

1. Cultivation of the cannabis plant carries a maximum penalty in a magistrates' court of a six-month prison sentence or a fine of £5000, or both, or, in a trial by jury, a 14-year prison sentence or an unlimited fine, or both.

The Misuse of Drugs Act 1971 prohibits particular activities in relation to 'controlled drugs' – these relate to the manufacture, possession and supply of certain drugs. The classification of drugs in Schedule 2 of this Act is based on the harm they may cause (see Table 13.1): class A, the most harmful, includes heroin and morphine; class B, of intermediate harm, includes amphetamines, codeine and cannabis (at the time of writing); and class C, the least harmful, includes steroids, most benzodiazepines and some hormones (Advisory Council on the Misuse of Drugs, 2002). The penalties applicable to the offences involving the different drugs are broadly related to these classifications. The Misuse of Drugs Regulations 2001 (Statutory Instrument 2001/ 3998) defines the categories of persons authorised in their professional capacities to supply and possess drugs controlled under the Act. In

Table 13.2 Summary of schedules of drugs set out in the Misuse of Drugs Regulations 2001

Schedule	Main drugs included	Restrictions
1	LSD, ecstasy, raw opium, psilocin, cannabis (herbal and resin)	Import, export, production, possession and supply only permitted under Home Office licence for medical or scientific research. Cannot be prescribed by doctors or dispensed by pharmacists
2	Heroin, cocaine, methadone, morphine, amphetamine, dexamphetamine, pethidine and quinalbarbitone	May be prescribed and lawfully possessed when on prescription. Otherwise, supply, possession, import, export and production are offences except under Home Office licence. Particular controls on their pre-scription, storage and record keeping apply
3	Barbiturates, temazepam, flunitrazepam, buprenorphine, pentazocine and diethylpropion	May be prescribed and lawfully possessed when on prescription. Otherwise, supply, possession, import, export and production are offences except under Home Office licence. Particular controls on their prescription and storage apply. Temazepam prescription requirements are less stringent than those for the other drugs in this Schedule
4 Part 1	Benzodiazepines (except flunitrazepam and temazepam) and pemoline	May be prescribed and lawfully possessed when on prescription. Otherwise, supply, possession, import, export and production are offences except under Home Office licence
4 Part 2	Anabolic steroids	May be lawfully possessed by anyone even without a prescription, provided they are in the form of a medical product
5	Compound preparations such as cough mixtures which contain small amounts of controlled drugs such as morphine. Some may be sold over the counter	Authority needed for their production or supply but can be freely imported, exported or possessed (without a prescription)

these Regulations the drugs are divided into five schedules, each specifying requirements governing such activities as export, supply, prescribing and record keeping (Table 13.2). The Misuse of Drugs Act and Regulations apply to adolescents and adults.

Right to education

Education is vital for the psychosocial development of the child and for equipping young people for an increasingly technological and skills-based economy. Education will enhance a young person's capacity for employment and ultimately to support a family. Non-attenders at school are more likely to be involved in crime and antisocial behaviour, and are more likely to be unemployed after leaving school. Furthermore, poor scholastic attainment is a risk factor for continued delinquency and drug misuse. Therefore, education has an important preventive role also.

In England, however, 50 000 children are out of school every day without good reason and, in particular, many substance-misusing young people are not at school. Some of these non-attenders will have been excluded. Yet Article 2 of the First Protocol of the Human Rights Act 1998, which gives effect to rights and freedoms guaranteed under the European Convention on Human Rights, records a right to education. It notes that 'no person shall be denied the right to education'. Article 28 of the United Nations Convention on the Rights of the Child also refers to the 'right of the child to education'. It could be argued that many of the most difficult and disadvantaged young people, often those at most risk of drug misuse, are in fact unable to exercise this right. Hence, to find a way of engaging these disaffected young people in education is an important challenge to schools, education authorities, communities and policy makers.

The Children Act 1989

The implementation of the Children Act was widely regarded as a significant improvement in the legislation regarding children. Some authorities described it as ground breaking in an international context. The major principles and concepts relevant to this subject may be set out as follows:

* The welfare of the child is paramount.
* The child's wishes and views must be considered.
* There should be minimum statutory intervention.
* There is a duty to safeguard and promote the welfare of the child.
* Agencies working with children should cooperate and work together in the best interests of the child.

Knowledge of the Children Act is key for those working with children and young people, who are not always served best by some of the well-meaning intentions of those more used to working with adults. Similarly, those working with children in need are not familiar with the ways in which drug-related issues may interact with child protection. This may be in relation to individual children or on a more organised basis, such as child prostitution.

Therefore it is essential to find the correct balance between engaging children and young people in appropriate services and not intervening inappropriately, while protecting children with the full weight of the law where needed. In order to achieve this it is necessary for professionals to receive adequate training and experience in working with children and their families, as well as in drug-related issues.

Working with other agencies is a cornerstone of work with children, and area child protection committees (ACPCs) play a central role in this. The ACPC can be used to coordinate and assist in producing coherent services that best meet the needs of children facing complex difficulties, as when both substance use and protection must be considered.

It is important to recognise that the wishes of the child, the parents and the service may be distinct from the best interests of the child. This delicate balance is often hard to find. However, in all cases the welfare of the child is paramount.

The Children Act makes it clear that the welfare of the child is the parents' responsibility. It is only under exceptional circumstances that there will be interference with this responsibility, by the action of the courts. This will be when a case has been made that parental responsibility must be shared, as in a care order; or where it is removed and given to different 'parents', as in adoption. These decisions are for the courts alone. Practitioners may play a role in giving evidence to the court but the decision is that of the judge.

It is good practice to ensure that parents both consent to and are involved in the assessment and treatment of their child. However, this may not be straightforward: for example, the child may object, a parent may be 'awkward', or there may be reasons to protect the child. In many senses, a need to protect the child is the easiest with which to deal logistically, as the guidelines for child protection drawn up by each ACPC should be followed. The welfare principle comes first. There is a need for openness with the parents and it is essential to work together in a multi-disciplinary context with statutory and other agencies (Department of Health, 1999).

In less extreme situations some principles can assist the clinician:

- The child should be actively encouraged to involve the parents.
- There can be some flexibility in the timing of parental involvement.
- It is possible to provide information without parental consent, at least in the beginning, when the time can be used to help the child to involve parents.
- It is adequate for a service to obtain the consent of only one parent, although it is better practice to have the consent of both.

- It is not necessary for parents to know the detailed content of treatment, even though they have given consent to it.

There are many skills available to clinicians working with children and adolescents that can assist in this difficult area. Generally recommended practice would be to involve one parent, or preferably both, whenever possible, and to respect the child's right to confidentiality, but with regard to the need to keep the child's welfare paramount. If, for example, a child gave the clinician information that required action, such as suicidal intent, then this must be shared so that the child can be kept safe and receive appropriate help.

Some services have expressed concern that if there is insistence on parental contact, the opportunity to help young substance users will be lost. If these situations cannot be ameliorated by using the principles stated above, then consideration of the child's competence becomes relevant. If there is a perceived risk to the child attendant upon involving the parents, child protection procedures may need to be invoked.

Competence and consent

With the exception of emergency life-saving treatment, which should be given as needed, the issue of consent by children to treatment is complex. Generally, those over the age of 18 years are regarded as adults and therefore competent to make decisions affecting their own welfare, including consent to their own medical treatment. Only where an adult is regarded as unable to assimilate and understand the information necessary to make such decisions, because of incapacity, are they regarded as incompetent. As a result of statute, young people between the ages of 16 and 18 years of age are usually regarded as competent, whereas those below the age of 16 years are generally treated as unable to give consent to their own medical treatment.

Parental responsibility lasts until the child is aged 18 years. However, the involvement of children in decisions deeply affecting them, such as treatment for drug misuse, will vary from child to child and family to family. To quote Lord Scarman:

'Parental rights yield to the child's right to make his own decisions when he reaches sufficient understanding and intelligence to be capable of making up his own mind on the matter requiring decision.'

Two other matters need consideration; the *parens patriae* doctrine, and the House of Lords *Gillick* ruling. Children (i.e. those under the age of 18 years) are subject to the *parens patriae* doctrine, which allows the court to make decisions on medical treatment in the child's best interests. This overrides any consent or refusal to treatment expressed by the child, the parents or anyone else.

The House of Lords' ruling in the case *Gillick* v. *West Norfolk and Wisbech Health Authority and the DHSS* (1986 AC112; 1985 3 WLR 830) permitted doctors to provide medical treatment to children without their parents' permission if they were under the age of 16 years but found by the doctor to be competent. In deciding whether a child is competent, a number of factors must be considered, as follows (British Medical Association & Law Society, 1995):

- ability to understand that there is a choice and that choices have consequences;
- willingness and ability to make a treatment decision, including the option of choosing that someone else makes that decision;
- understanding of the nature and purpose of the proposed procedure;
- understanding of the risks and side-effects of the proposed procedure;
- understanding of the alternatives to the proposed procedure and the risks attached to them, and the consequences of no treatment;
- freedom from pressure.

There is little doubt that later case law has modified the effect of the *Gillick* ruling, and certainly the younger the child the less likely it is that the child will be found competent to consent to medical treatment. There is serious doubt as to whether some drug-using children could be regarded as competent to give consent to treatment without a parent's agreement. There is also a body of legal opinion that advises that many children under the age of 13 or 14 years would not be regarded as competent to consent to medical treatment for drug misuse without the involvement of their parents (Dale-Perera & Hamilton, 1997).

Treatment without consent

While adults cannot be legally compelled under the Mental Health Act 1983 to have treatment against their will unless they are severely mentally ill, a child can be compelled to have treatment if a court thinks it is necessary. Thus, if the court decides that it is in the best interests of the child, it may overrule the wishes of the child and parents. This has been done in relation to eating disorders, religious objections to blood transfusions and life-saving surgery.

There has been little use of the Mental Health Act 1983 in relation to children with complex disorders involving mental health. However, a new Mental Health Act is proposed, under which it is possible that more children and young people will be assessed and treated. The debate about this is wide ranging. It includes concerns about the stigmatisation of children who have been 'sectioned'. Also, if they are not detained with all the safeguards that are part of the proposed Act, then there is the possibility of infringement of their human rights. This matter is of particular importance where there is concern about the mental health of a young person who may be misusing drugs.

How much can be done without parental consent? As noted previously, Lord Scarman has emphasised that good practice requires practitioners 'to consult parents and guardians and to obtain their consent to, and involvement in, the treatment of young people'. Therefore, the issue is not whether parents should be involved, but rather the timing of such involvement. Generally, with support over time, many children and young people can be helped to involve their parents. If this is totally refused and there is a risk of losing contact with the young person, then how far a service can go in providing intervention must be considered. Generally, the lower the level of intervention, the less stringent will be the need to comply with high levels of capacity to consent by the young person.

Perhaps the lowest level of intervention is the giving of information. Drug education must be sensible and accurate and conform to accepted professional opinion. Many would accept that such information could be given without parental consent. However, it is worth considering that many schools seek parental consent before giving sex education, and sometimes religious education, to pupils.

Drug prevention may encompass activities that range from giving information and advice on how to refuse drugs, to offering a needle exchange. Some would argue that offering needle exchanges constitutes treatment. The liability of those providing premises for this activity, such as a school or youth club, is far from clear.

Counselling would be considered by many to be a form of treatment. Capacity to consent is therefore relevant here, and it may be wise to bear in mind experience from the debate about false memory syndrome (ideas may be implanted in children and young people's minds). It is likely that to provide prescriptions to someone under the age of 16 years without parental consent is ill advised. Where parents withhold such consent unreasonably, the involvement of social services, and possibly the courts, may be relevant. Private prescribing of substitute drugs is strongly discouraged (Royal College of Psychiatrists & Royal College of Physicians, 2000).

Confidentiality

In considering issues of confidentiality, the guiding principle is what is in the best interests of the child. It should be noted that there is no time-scale to such an imperative – it is an abiding principle. While it may be important to be able to engage the young person in order for professionals to help, no blanket assurance of confidentiality should be given, as it may be impossible to maintain this. The guidance given by Lord Scarman is important:

'It is good practice to consult parents and guardians and to obtain their consent to, and involvement in, the treatment of young people.' (Royal College of Psychiatrists, 1987).

The most important issue to require a breach of any assurance of confidentiality is when a child is at risk of harm. A service that maintains confidentiality in these circumstances must bear in mind the risk of future claims of negligence if the child is harmed as a result of failure to share information. Such an action could be brought by parents who were not enabled to protect their child as a result of lack of information, or by a child who was exposed to risk or actually harmed. A child may bring an action many years after the event. A statutory authority charged with the care of a child may act as a 'litigation friend' and bring an action on behalf of a child.

Consider also the situation where the child or young person may give information not only about their own drug use, but also that of others and methods of supply. If some of these activities take place in a school, for example, and place others at risk, lack of information sharing may lead to litigation by the school or other children or parents. Thus, far from acting in the best interests of the child, a service or individual who fails to disclose sensitive information may be considered as colluding in situations that expose a child to risk.

Risk of significant harm

'Significant harm' is a term used in the Children Act and is generally taken to mean harm that is worthy of legal note. Evidence as to whether a child is suffering, or is likely to suffer, significant harm must be evaluated when a young person is assessed. This harm may arise directly from the drug use, from involvement in crime or prostitution or other forms of exploitation, or from the context within which the drug use began. The harm could result from, for example, an unhappy and possibly abusive family life, mental illness and other multiple complex difficulties interacting with adverse results.

It is necessary to consider the difficult issue of parents who are drug users. A serious drug misuse problem on the part of parents can have serious consequences for the lives of their children (Davis, 1990; Keen & Alison, 2001). Whereas there is no evidence that all parents who use illegal drugs are incapable of caring for their children, this is a matter that must be raised for some families. In the same way that it is good practice for those working with children to ask about family factors, including drug use, so those working with adults should make enquiries about the welfare of children.

The idea of a child 'in need' is also useful in working with drug-misusing children. Very often there are multiple problems not only for the child but also for the carers. The identification of a child 'in need' alerts professionals to this, and can sometimes produce assistance from professional and voluntary agencies that is highly valued. Unfortunately, with few resources available, it is most likely that these will be directed at those identified as at greater risk of harm. The opportunity for any preventive work, even at an advanced level, is missed.

Thus the concepts of risk and significant harm are of great importance to those working with children and young people who are misusing drugs. The greater the assessment of risk of harm, the greater will be the need to involve parents and other agencies. One difficulty is the lack of standard practice for the assessment of risk. Another problem is the lack of work with other agencies involved in child care, even at an anonymous consultation level. Experience in working with the statutory agencies involved in child protection is very helpful in dealing with this difficult area and is certainly a practice guideline for those trying to help children and young people (Department of Health, 1999; Murphy & Oulds, 2000).

Practice issues

There are some strategies to facilitate practice in this area. The development of clear guidelines, for instance for assessment, including the assessment of competence, as well as for clinical decision-making, could standardise practice and provide a reliable service approach for those who use them. Guidelines also permit audit and monitoring of practice and, if complied with, provide protection for practitioners (for example against claims of malpractice). In working with children and young people who misuse drugs it is sensible to look at the practices of other agencies working with children facing difficulties, such as the ACPCs.

Children are entitled to a high standard of practice. Thus, meaningful accountability is necessary and this must pervade all areas of practice, including accurate and full keeping of notes, and supervision and training. There is sometimes debate about keeping notes, but it is worth considering that if no notes are kept, there is little recourse to justice for either the child or the service. Litigation could be a matter of one person's word against another's.

There is sometimes debate about the role of consultation provided by one service to another or one individual to a service. One expectation is that all participants should be responsible within the roles and limits of their expertise. If people providing consultation find that this is not so, they must consider their responsibility to prevent serious harm to vulnerable individuals. The same responsibility extends to 'whistle blowing'.

Conclusions

There are a number of legal and ethical issues to be considered in structuring services for drug-misusing young people. It must be acknowledged that breach of confidentiality is an ethical problem for many workers in this field. The principle of doing at least some good may be a convincing argument. However, the proposition that a little good will result, at least in the short term, is untested. Against this must be put the weight of accumulated experience of managing these matters according to legal principles. There also should be some acknowledgement that a large group of experienced practitioners has found that these principles do work in the best interests of children, and that each of us at different times will undoubtedly be wrong. Against this background the following issues may be considered:

- Practitioners need to have a clear knowledge about the legal framework and experience in working within it. Acknowledgement that the legal imperatives for work with children differ from those applied to adults is essential. The guiding principle that the welfare of the child is paramount must be applied in all approaches to this work.
- There must be recognition of the roles and responsibilities of parents in work with children and young people.
- There is a duty to deliver the best possible services to these vulnerable young people and a need to keep their best interests at the heart of this practice, whether in the statutory or voluntary sector.
- All services should be accountable for their work and every method necessary to enable this should be continually employed. There is a responsibility for all services not only to ensure best practice but also to indemnify services and their employees against legal challenge.
- Consideration should be given to learning from other services involved in work with needy young people. Recognition that there are common problems leads to less professional isolation and fewer unusual practices. If there is a reason to deviate from a statutory requirement or guidelines, this must be clearly explained and recorded. All agencies and individuals must recognise that they are responsible and accountable for what they do, and unusual practice may not only harm the children they work with but may lead to litigation, even at some distant date.
- There is a responsibility for all services not only to ensure best practice but also to provide insurance against legal challenge, so that if financial compensation is needed it can be provided.

- Services for young people who misuse drugs need to be part of wider service provision for children, and to this end membership of a local ACPC is worth considering. This would ensure that drug and children's services work together within jointly accepted guidelines, train together, and identify and deal with problems that arise together. Some shared professional culture could enhance collaborative practice, especially if there is regular access to discussion and legal advice and the opportunity to shape services in the best interests of children and young people. The ability to argue coherently and to demonstrate a high level of professionalism is an asset in the advocacy role and in service delivery in general.

That which is legal may well not be ethical, but a good knowledge of both is required.

Acknowledgements

Many thanks to Sarah Woolrich, barrister, for her helpful comments, and to Sue Mitchell and Chris Kottler at the Home Office for their advice relating to the Misuse of Drugs Act.

References

Advisory Council on the Misuse of Drugs (2002) *The Classification of Cannabis Under the Misuse of Drugs Act 1971*. London: Home Office.

Association of Police Surgeons & Royal College of Psychiatrists (2000) *Substance Misuse Detainees in Police Custody* (Council Report CR81). London: Royal College of Psychiatrists.

British Medical Association & Law Society (1995) *Assessment of Mental Capacity: Guidance for Doctors and Lawyers*. London: British Medical Association.

Dale-Perera, A. & Hamilton, C. (1997) *An Outline of Some of the Key Issues Raised During the Development of National Policy Guidelines on Working with Young Drug Users*. London: Children's Legal Centre.

Davis, S. (1990) Chemical dependency in women: a description of effects and outcome on adequate parenting. *Journal of Substance Abuse and Treatment*, **7**, 225–232.

Department of Health (1999) *Working Together to Safeguard Children: A Guide to Inter-agency Working to Safeguard and Promote the Welfare of Children*. London: Department of Health.

Gilvarry, E., Christian, J., Crome, I., *et al* (2001) *The Substance of Young Needs*. London: Health Advisory Service .

Keen, J. & Alison, L. (2001) Drug misusing parents: key points for health professionals. *Archives of Disease in Childhood*, **85**, 296–299.

Lord Scarman (1999) In *Child Psychiatry and the Law* (eds D. Black, S. Wolkind & J. Harris-Hendricks), p. 100. London: Gaskell.

Murphy, M. & Oulds, G. (2000) Establishing and developing co-operative links between substance misuse and child protection systems. In *Substance Misuse and Childcare: How to Understand, Assist and Intervene When Drugs Affect Parenting* (eds F. Harbin & M. Murphy), pp. 111–122. Lyme Regis: Russell House.

Royal College of Psychiatrists (1987) Confidentiality: current concerns of child and adolescent psychiatric teams. *Bulletin of the Royal College of Psychiatrists*, **11**, 170–171.

—— & Royal College of Physicians (2000) *Drugs: Dilemmas and Choices*. London: Gaskell.

CHAPTER 14

Developing an evidence-based model for services

Richard Williams, Eilish Gilvarry and Jane Christian

Key points

- Evidence-based service design should bring together strategic leadership and management, policy, awareness of equity gaps, the views of users and carers, the clinical realities and the research evidence.
- Its aims, objectives and principles should underpin a client-based approach.
- Services should recognise the high levels of comorbidity of substance misuse, psychiatric disorder, and many other health, education and social problems for young people.
- Broad, well-articulated, multi-disciplinary and multi-agency services should be responsive to the real needs of children, young people and their carers and the growing awareness of the common pathways to substance misuse.
- The strategic framework recommended in this chapter comprises all four tiers of health care.
- The organisational culture, therapeutic environments, collaboration and workforce sustainment and development must be right.

Components of a successful service model

Policy and strategy

Developing a model for any public sector service requires a lead from policy, and clear statements of the strategic intent and direction for the service relating to an identified client group. These considerations should evoke the aims, objectives and principles that underpin the design and delivery of the service. When combined with evidence about need, supply, demand and service effectiveness, and the opinions of users, carers and practitioners, these strategic statements allow planners to prioritise service developments. In other words, the model should draw on *evidence-based policy*, and *evidence-based and values-based practice* (Fulford and Williams, 2003) to marry critical aspects of vision, values and planning with research evidence, the clinical realities and child-centredness, to help us to develop services that are appropriate, realistic, effective and capable of further evolution.

Evidence on need, supply, demand and effectiveness

Need, supply and demand are linked as a dynamic trio of forces. This book shows that the current level of need for substance misuse services is high and that it greatly outstrips the capacity of services to respond. A review by Barton *et al* (2002) provides an entry point to the literature on children's mental health, risk and service effectiveness. Bushell *et al* (2002) produced a literature review relating to substance misuse. A wide array of interventions could be delivered but presently there are substantial imbalances between the resources available, particularly well-trained staff, and demands for services. This is just the kind of situation in which increases in service provision will provoke further demand.

A successful service model must recognise these and other system dynamics. It must balance perceptions of need, as seen by professionals, with the opinions and expectations of potential clients (Buston, 2002), but be realistically informed by present service capacities and capabilities and the realities of clinical practice. The client group anticipated for the service should be explicitly acknowledged by the model, which, if mature and appropriate, should enable priority setting according to explicit criteria. The priorities chosen should be tempered by evidence of effectiveness of interventions from research that must not exclude clients with complex problems, who are likely to need the very services that are the subject of this chapter.

A strategic framework

In order to bring all of the foregoing considerations together, a service model requires a strategic framework that should support purposeful negotiation of the roles of the various components of the service and effective communications with related services.

Workforce and organisational development plans

An effective service model should have the flexibility to underpin the implementation of services and enable development of the organisations that provide them. Above all, it must be practical and take on board the vital matters of workforce recruitment, retention and development in a planned way that is appropriate to the skills required of the service. The issues arising for practitioners from working in a world that is complex and uncertain have been identified elsewhere (Williams, 2002). The model must take them on. Likewise, it should recognise the importance to success of getting right organisational culture and, therefore, contain an organisational development plan.

Evidence-based service design

Evidence-based service design (EBSD) describes a method of planning services that endeavours to deal with each of the items summarised so far, and this chapter illustrates it by developing a model for commissioning and delivering services for young people who use or misuse substances. Appropriately, EBSD draws on evidence from research and clinical practice but a wide range of other sources too, and the standards of evidence include but are not restricted to those of clinical science (Barton *et al*, 2002; Edwards *et al*, 2002). By way of illustration, we bring additional evidence together with summaries of key issues from previous

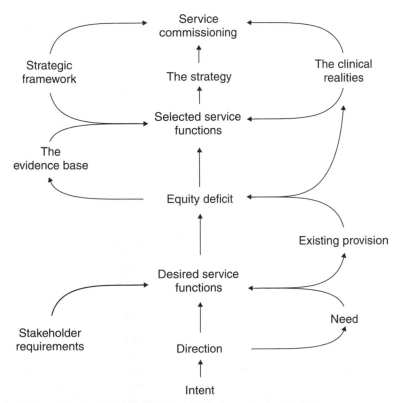

Figure 14.1 A mechanism for designing and commissioning services.

chapters to establish a reasoned model for commissioning and delivering services for young people who use or misuse substances. Figure 14.1 summarises these processes in creating strategy and commissioning services.

The aims, objectives and principles of services

Current UK policy emphasises young people and communities; it focuses on making education and treatment more available to young people, particularly vulnerable young people. UK policy on responses to and interventions to prevent substance misuse is formed increasingly by awareness of the risk factors (Barton & Quinn, 2001; Bushell *et al*, 2002). The government has been congratulated for the consistency of its policies and for its basis in evidence rather than rhetoric (Farrell & Strang, 1998).

Aims

Necessarily, the aims for services for young people who use or misuse substances must be broad but sufficiently specific to give clarity about what is required and the way forward. The aims listed below are based on *The Substance of Young Needs* (Williams *et al*, 1996), the review of that work by the Health Advisory Service in 2000–01 (Gilvarry *et al*, 2001), and policy. They include:

- to provide a broad range of services that are sufficient to offer effective responses to young people who have health, social and education problems that arise from or are associated with substance use or misuse, with the intention of alleviating those problems and reducing social exclusion and its consequences;
- to provide longer-term approaches to substance use and misuse, with the intention of promoting the developmental, health, social and educational well-being of young people, with a view to reducing risk, increasing resilience and contributing to the longer-term health and well-being of the population most at risk;
- to provide very specialised services that are of sufficient capacity and capability to respond effectively to those young people in serious need;
- to work in partnerships with young people, their families and all relevant services in the statutory and non-statutory sectors.

Objectives

In order to achieve these ambitious aims, services should have clear objectives. Suggestions are given in Box 14.1.

Box 14.1 Service objectives

- To involve young people, their parents and their carers in a meaningful way in planning, commissioning and delivering services.
- To establish child-centred services that take into account the views of young people and their families.
- To provide effective and timely interventions for young people who present with problems arising from substance use or misuse.
- To make services equitably available, according to need.
- To provide sufficient general and specialist services to enable a full range of functions to be discharged.
- To provide well-integrated services that can contribute positively to: increasing social inclusion; early recognition, assessment, and intervention with psychiatric disorders; early recognition and assessment of, and intervention with, specific substance misuse syndromes.
- To provide services that are able to manage demand and meet projected increases in demand in timely and effective ways.
- To offer services that are based on sound evidence but open to new ideas.
- To encourage an environment in which research can flourish and be properly assessed and disseminated.
- To promote a multi-agency, multi-disciplinary approach and integrated service provision that works across the boundaries between departments within agencies, and sectors of care.
- To build into all services child protection measures that provide safeguards for children and young people wherever and whenever they are cared for or treated.
- To link with other programmes on social exclusion, substance misuse, mental health and offending.
- To reduce the stigma surrounding use of services for young people who misuse substances.
- To cultivate an atmosphere of mutual support among professionals, academics, managers and the public across the statutory and non-statutory sector services.
- To draw on and disseminate good practice.

The principles of a developmental approach

In order to deliver the aims and objectives we sketch here, a number of key principles should underpin commissioning and delivery. Each develops the objectives in more detail.

Everybody's Business, the strategy for child and adolescent mental health services in Wales (National Assembly for Wales, 2001), advances eight items as general principles. *The Substance of Young Needs* (Williams *et al*, 1996) described ten key principles for services for young people who use and misuse substances and, later, the Children's Legal Centre and the Standing Conference on Drug Abuse published a follow-up to that report with its own adaptation of those principles (Dale-Perera *et al*, 1999). Combining these three approaches, we offer eight broad principles. They are that services should be:

- child-centred;
- protective of children and adolescents;
- respectful of parental responsibility and lawful;
- equitable and appropriate;
- competent and responsive;
- accountable and espouse further development of good practice;
- holistic;
- efficient, effective and targeted.

Each of these principles could be developed to generate standards against which success should be reviewed. For example, it is axiomatic that a model of services for young people should be orientated to the needs, preferences, lifestyles and culture of young people. This requires developmentally oriented and child-centred approaches. Children and adolescents change dramatically as they grow and develop across the first two decades of life, and services for them should be appropriate to their circumstances and developmental maturity at every relevant age. Child and adolescent mental health services should provide good

---

Box 14.2 Child-centred services

Child-centredness means focusing on:
- childrens' rights (consistent with the United Nations Convention on the Rights of the Child);
- paramountcy of children's welfare;
- provision of advocacy services;
- provision of child-friendly services;
- active steps to hear the voices of children.

This requires professionals to:
- view each child as a developing person in his or her own context;
- view problems in the ways in which children experience them;
- include a focus on prevention and health promotion;
- develop relationships that aid young people to tackle their problems realistically.

The model should take into account:
- the developmental stages of all children and adolescents who may use the service;
- the cultural background, age, gender and readiness to change of children and their families;
- the evidence base on interventions in age-appropriate environments;
- the assessment and management of multiple areas of functioning;
- the importance of family involvement when intervening.

---

examples, and there is no reason to think that services for young people who use and misuse substances should be based on different general principles. Box 14.2 (developed from *Everybody's Business*) lists the properties of child-centred services.

However, many young people experience deprivation and social exclusion. These matters have to be grasped by our model if services are to be appropriately oriented to the client group, because of their powerful links (both by way of cause and effect) with substance misuse. The Carlile review (National Assembly for Wales, 2002), which gives an agenda for designers of all children's services, shows what can go wrong for very needy young people when services are insufficiently child-centred. Buston (2002) identifies the further work to be done by practitioners in our current child and adolescent mental health services to achieve effective communication skills.

Need

There are several ways in which need may be characterised. In the National Health Service (NHS), *comparative* assessments benchmark services in an area against those in similar areas on the basis of epidemiological studies of morbidity, the services provided and their use, outcomes and costs. *Corporate* assessments combine comparative methods with local information from users, carers and providers. However, 'needs assessment' has a different meaning within UK local government. It describes the needs of individuals, and these are often set against eligibility criteria. The new Assessment Framework established by the government in England and Wales (Department of Health *et al*, 2000; National Assembly for Wales and Home Office, 2001) illustrates this approach.

Equity deficits

The notion of an equity deficit is attributable to the work of Warner & Furnish (2002), who described the concept with reference to Alzheimer's disease. In the case of young substance misusers, policy recommends providing enhanced services for this group in need, but to identify the requirements for service development of that population, it is important to know where, and in what ways, the levels of service are lacking. Mapping services that are assisting or even deterring substance misusers from gaining access to interventions from which they might benefit will identify gaps in provision and the steps to be taken towards filling the 'equity deficit' through a 'heightened equality of concern'.

What is key in Warner & Furnish's approach to need is that it identifies gaps not only in provision directly related to substance misuse but also in those services that impact upon the factors that influence substance misuse, including people's lifestyles, circumstances and non-health needs. Earlier chapters have surveyed the roles of a wide range of factors in order better to understand the origins and conse-quences of substance misuse and the decisions made by young people to become involved or not. The available evidence supports the equity deficit approach, as recent effectiveness research tentatively suggests that approaches that solely target symptoms or syndromes are in-sufficient, while those that also take on the risk factors are more effective (Brown *et al*, 2001; Grella *et al*, 2001).

Definitions of use and misuse

When designing services, it is important to be clear about the meanings of the terms that are used, as the scope and nature of the services stem from these definitions. But it was apparent to the NHS Health Advisory Service (Williams & Richardson, 1995) during the course of its fieldwork in 1994 that there was wide variation in the terminology in use. Recently, one of us (R.W.) has been responsible for fieldwork to consider need in south-east Wales, where the research has found persisting uncertainty about definitions (Byrne *et al*, 2002). In part, this seems to reflect confusion between definitions that are used for research and classification purposes, and definitions of the often complex needs of the client groups that are found in practice. As this chapter is concerned with service design, the definitions used endeavour to include all who might be referred to and benefit from comprehensive services.

We adopt Dale-Perera *et al's* (1999) definition of 'substance' as being 'Any psychotropic substance, including illegal drugs, illicit use of prescription drugs and volatile substances'. Dale-Perera *et al* argue that 'young people's drug taking should not be considered in isolation from alcohol and volatile substances'. We include tobacco, too, because of the amounts that young people consume, its harm and addictiveness, and the compounding effects it can have on use of other drugs. For example, drug use (largely cannabis) has been found to be higher among smokers, and tobacco and alcohol consumption have an association with later drug use (Miller & Plant, 1996).

We concur with the opinion of the NHS Health Advisory Service that clear distinctions between use and misuse are hard to draw:

'Most drug use is illegal and some who use and experiment may have adverse consequences, sometimes fatal. However, use of alcohol safely in the older adolescent cannot be considered misuse. We recognise that use of substances has different implications at different ages.' (Williams *et al*, 1996)

Drugscope refers to 'drug taking'. It acknowledges that harm can occur through use, whether through intoxication, legal or health problems.

In this chapter, we employ the term *use* to describe ingestion of a pharmacologically active substance that does not appear to produce any consequential or associated developmental, social, educational or health harm. We take *misuse* to encompass the definitions of harmful use, dependence and use that are part of a wider spectrum of problematic or harmful behaviour (Williams *et al*, 1996). Following the line taken by the NHS Health Advisory service, for the purpose of service design, misuse is a broad category. For example, young people might be described as misusing substances when they are not suffering pharmacological harm attributable to a substance, but when their use is part of, or contributes to, a wider spectrum of problems that may lie in developmental, social or educational arenas.

Perhaps as confirmation, Aarons *et al* (2001) showed that young people in receipt of substance misuse services also receive assistance from other services, including youth justice, mental health and school services for emotional, behavioural and child welfare problems. It is also possible that a young person has no such problems when misuse describes harm to health through dependence, addiction or another substance use disorder.

Prevalence

There have been many estimates of the levels of substance use and misuse by young people and summaries of recent findings are provided in earlier chapters. Weinberg *et al* (1998) reviewed and synthesised the literature on adolescent substance misuse, covering natural history, epidemiology, aetiology, comorbidity, assessment, treatment and prevention.

There are tendencies both to over- and to underestimate, as a result of the methodologies used and the sensitivity and publicity attached to the subject. The majority of the statistics available are estimations based upon the responses of young people who present for treatment or who answer self-report surveys, and a significant difficulty in assessing patterns of use and misuse arises from using school-based samples. Some of these surveys leave out truants and excluded students, but they are often the ones most at risk (Goulden & Sondhi, 2001).

While we conclude that the levels of substance use and misuse by young people are high, there remain problems in getting a clear picture of actual needs based on prevalence studies. Some are due to the diverse effects of substance misuse and others result from the many fears of adults regarding stigma, losing the care of their children and penalisation by the authorities.

Risk and resilience

Chapter 4 summarises the determinants of substance misuse and Chapter 6 deals with the overlapping risk and resilience factors for substance misuse and psychiatric disorder in young people (Box 14.3 provides an evidence-based summary).

There is a broad range of experiences that contribute to social disadvantage and deprivation, including health, education and economic hardship, poor access to services, poor transport and low community cohesion. Barton *et al* (2002) and Juang & Silbereisen (2002) provide additional evidence. In 2001, the UK government defined social exclusion as follows:

'A short-hand term for what can happen when people or areas suffer from a combination of problems such as unemployment, poor skills, low incomes, poor housing, high crime environment, bad health and family breakdown.' (Social Exclusion Unit, 2001)

Tudor Hart's Inverse Care Law (1971) still applies, and there is evidence that inequity is often mediated through carers.

Consequently, certain young people are more at risk than others of misusing substances. There is now abundant evidence that young people who experience social exclusion are more likely to use and misuse substances. In particular, substance use rises in line with the levels of: truancy and school exclusion; criminal activity; homelessness and runaways; and living with a family whose members use drugs.

Box 14.3 Risk and resilience factors for substance misuse and psychiatric disorder

Risk factors
- The number of exposures to risk rather than the specific types of risk.
- Low socio-economic status.
- Poverty.
- Family instability and conflict.
- Maltreatment.
- Poor parenting.
- Problems with attachment patterns.
- Parental psychopathology and substance misuse.

Resilience factors
- Positive temperament.
- Intellectual ability.
- Supportive family.
- Encouraging and rewarding social support system.
- A good, caring relationship with at least one adult.

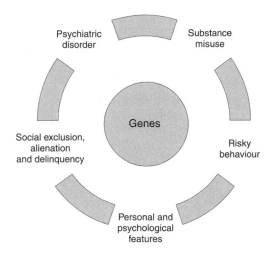

Figure 14.2 Circular relationships between factors bearing on substance misuse.

Other vulnerable groups include young people who are looked after and those with mental disorders. Government policy considers them all to be priorities (Central Drugs Coordination Unit, 1999; National Assembly for Wales, 2000*a,b*).

Recent research on adolescents (aged 10–16 years) (Giancola & Parker, 2001) has highlighted particular personal factors as predictors of substance misuse. These risk factors include problems with executive functioning and temperament (e.g. cognitive disabilities that include poor organisational skills and poor abstract reasoning, and hyperactivity, irritability, poor attention levels and poor reaction to stimuli withdrawal). While that research noted that peer relationships and aggressive behaviour featured on a pathway to drug use, it recognised that psychiatric risk factors were most significant in predicting higher levels of drug use.

Conversely, the American Academy of Pediatrics Commission on Substance Misuse (2001) argues that antisocial behaviour is the product of substance misuse. Bonomo *et al* (2001) apply Becker's (1991) sociological theory of labelling in deviant subcultures to explain that labelling people as deviant reinforces their behaviour as part of their identity, and so contributes to a spiral of decline into the label. We conclude that the consequences of substance misuse and psychiatric disorder are similar to the risk factors and include greater vulnerability and social exclusion.

There are very strong indicators now of the significance of genetic factors to childhood mental health problems and disorders. While some genes relate to specific disorders, it is probable that most generally affect the vulnerability and resilience of children and young people.

Also, it is likely that there is an independent genetic effect mediated through the effects of genes on personality and temperament (Goldberg, 2002). Furthermore, there is now substantial opinion that environmental factors determine whether or not and to what degree genetic factors affect individuals.

This review, taken together with the review by Bushell *et al* (2002), suggests the circular framework of relationships depicted in Figure 14.2.

Comorbidity

Chapter 6 summarises what is known about the comorbidity of substance misuse with psychiatric conditions. A review by Barton *et al* (2002) provides a summary of some research evidence.

Bonomo *et al* (2001) argue that while psychiatric disorder makes substance misuse more likely, the combination of substance misuse with psychiatric disorder can result in higher levels of risky behaviour than would be present without comorbidity. In other words, psychological and psychiatric risk factors need to be understood in terms of their contribution to substance misuse, but also their implications once combined with substance misuse. The co-occurrence of developmental, health, education and social problems is higher in substance users than in non-users and, as Zeitlin (1999) argues, the 'comorbid condition' is compounded by 'vulnerability, lack of family protection and exposure to a source of drugs'.

We highlight three matters. First, finding high levels of comorbidity is not surprising, as substance misuse, psychiatric disorders and many other health problems – as well as lower use of services, and education and social problems – share overlapping risk and resilience factors. The triad of deprivation and poverty, psychiatric disorder and substance misuse holds together. Recent studies investigating longitudinal predictors of drug use claim that the concurrent existence of social exclusion and psychiatric disorder provides a pathway to substance misuse (Kuperman *et al*, 2001; Mullen & Barry, 2001; Pedersen *et al*, 2001). Ferdinand *et al* (2001) claim that risk factors can develop in a chain, to form a pathway that may first involve peer relationships, then delinquent behaviour, and finally drug use. Social exclusion and psychiatric disorders can also be the cause of non-recognition of substance misuse, comorbidity and non-attendance at services.

Second, comorbidity is a professional concept that describes the many situations in which single syndromes do not adequately describe the common experiences and needs of the population at risk. However, patients/clients do not see or experience their problems as disjointed in this way.

Third, the significance of comorbidity to professional practice and EBSD is that it emphasises the importance of viewing people's needs from a broad perspective and providing articulated services that are able to respond to the real and interconnected needs of the public. Indicative findings from several recent studies show that where only substance misuse is treated, comorbid behavioural conditions re-emerge in conjunction with higher levels of substance use after treatment to a greater extent than in non-comorbid youths (Brown *et al*, 2001; Grella *et al*, 2001).

The service developments required

The approach

The evidence shows that the health care needs of young people who misuse substances should not be considered in isolation from their other needs, and that service delivery should be approached from a multi-agency, child-centred, yet family-oriented perspective (Spoth *et al*, 2001; National Assembly for Wales, 2002). Indications are that interventions that address risk factors alongside substance misuse can be more successful than other approaches (Rivers *et al*, 2001). Focusing on social roles, harm reduction, flexibility in delivery and a client-led approach, with counselling available to cover a range of areas, including substances, provides a framework for tackling risk factors and substance misuse simultaneously.

The core service functions in our model are: education, prevention, intervention and training. Education includes providing young people with accurate and well-founded information, working with their attitudes, and support to enable their acquisition of greater social skills so that they are able to make purposeful choices and avoid substance use. The aims of prevention are to promote resilience and tackle risk factors that may propel young people who are using substances to progress to misuse. There are important lessons for designers of education and prevention programmes from the widely differing assessments of future risk of misuse by users and non-users (Sutherland & Shepherd, 2002).

In the USA, education and prevention programmes are defined by their audience (see Chapter 2). *Universal programmes* are intended to reach the general population (e.g. school-based education programmes) and should be comprehensive, with well-coordinated components for individuals, families and communities. *Selective programmes* target people who are at high risk (e.g. children of adults who use substances); those that deliver a range of individual and family-based interventions have resulted in significant reductions in problem behaviour (e.g. Kumpfer *et al*, 1996). *Indicated programmes* (e.g. Reconnecting Youth) deliver a range of interventions that are aimed at individuals, their peer groups and their families. They address many domains of functioning (Eggert *et al*, 1994; Sussman, 1996) and are designed for young people who have already used drugs and show disruptive behaviours (Belcher & Schinitzly, 1998).

The intervention services are those that offer assessment, treatment and other appropriate activities to young people who have problems arising from their use of substances, whether they lie within diagnosable disorder or wider social and educational realms. Therefore, they include a range of psychiatric, medical and psychological assessments and treatments.

Box 14.4 Professional opinion in South Wales about service development

Orientation of services
Most addiction services are configured for adults. Services for younger people should be tailored to local patterns of substance use and misuse by young people.

Age range
The age range of young people who may require services continues to extend. This has provoked demand for education, prevention and interventions that are appropriate for children. The age range of young people as defined by government policy (up to 25 years) is too broad for practical service design, as it covers children, young adolescents, older adolescents and young adults who may well be parents. Young people should be split into age groups (e.g. up to 15, 16–17 and 18–25 years).

Filling gaps in services
Requirements include: increased provision of core services oriented to younger people; better family support services; services for children and young people whose parents/carers misuse substances; advocacy services; and better availability of high-quality educational materials.

Training
There are big gaps in training available to people who work with children and young people.

Integration of services
Greater integration of primary care, mental health, child and school health, education, social and addiction services is required, as are: better definition of the roles of the various agencies; clear referral systems; unambiguous pathways and partnerships across agencies; and common systems for data collection and information sharing.

Funding
Funds for services for young people who use or misuse substances should be ring-fenced, integrated across agencies and support long-term developments.

Ascertainment of local requirements for service development

Already, this extraction of the evidence has created a huge agenda for service development, but tuning it to the local circumstances is another key part of EBSD. Dale-Perera *et al* (1999) agree that local knowledge is crucial to needs assessment. This requires ethnographic research in each area (e.g. that conducted through focus groups and interviews with professionals, the agencies involved and young people) to provide a localised picture of the equity deficits of young substance users and gaps in service that require attention.

We illustrate this advice by extracting information from the corporate needs assessment of services required by young people in south-east Wales who use or misuse substances, conducted between 2000 and 2002. Around 40 professionals from a wide range of disciplines and services were interviewed and all had in common the likelihood of coming into contact with young people at risk of substance misuse. This qualitative enquiry revealed common concerns about the capability and capacity of local services and a broad consensus of opinion about key issues that should influence service design (Box 14.4) (Byrne *et al*, 2002).

The clinical realities

Young people most frequently use tobacco, alcohol or cannabis. Anecdotally, the prevalence of misuse of prescribed drugs is higher in some places than previously estimated and use of so-called 'hard' drugs increases with age, from low levels comparative to alcohol misuse early in adolescence to rather more substantial levels, particularly after the age of 18.

Most young people who misuse substances also have problems that lie in the wider domains described earlier. A smaller but very needy group aged under 18 years are those who use substances chaotically, and they appear to have especially high levels of social exclusion and alienation. A rather smaller group of young people are affected by substance use syndromes that are appropriately described within ICD–10 or DSM–IV (see Chapter 1), and a minority of young people require specialised addiction services. Very many more young people have psychiatric disorder that is comorbid with their substance misuse.

The Substance of Young Needs (Williams *et al*, 1996), the NHS Health Advisory Service's report of a thematic review of the requirements for and availability of services for young people who misuse substances, concluded that services were ad hoc, extremely thin, unrelated to need, provided mainly by the non-statutory sector and poorly coordinated. It found pockets of isolated excellence but, strikingly, huge equity deficits.

Since then, as a result of a spur from policy and growing professional investment in the field, there has been some development of services for young people, although, anecdotally, the effects have been reported to be patchy, and this has occurred alongside little evaluation, particularly with regard to outcome. Developmentally appropriate services include primary, secondary and tertiary programmes of intervention but some have little theoretical basis (Winters, 1999). Readers will have noted from earlier chapters that there is actually a substantial body of evidence on theory and effectiveness.

Present community programmes range from self-help groups, through school-based counselling, to structured activities as more appropriate alternatives to substance use. Where specialist out-patient addiction services are presently available, they usually provide brief contact with trained professionals and, too often, intervention in single functional areas. We know of only one area in England in which in-patient beds are provided specifically for adolescents dependent on alcohol and drugs who require admission for their safe detoxification.

User preferences

Another dimension of the work undertaken in south-east Wales (Byrne *et al*, 2002) consisted of focus groups run with children and adolescents in three age groups, from 12 to 18 years, in schools but also, importantly, in other community facilities to ensure contact with excluded and truanting young people, who are at higher risk.

This showed that the majority of young people had a reasonably sophisticated knowledge of the subject and opinions that reflected the public debate on drugs and alcohol. Typically, the young people tended to underestimate the dangers of alcohol, despite the vast majority knowing at least one person who had been hospitalised as a result of it. The young people gave estimates of prevalence and availability of substances that match recent surveys.

It appeared that use of drugs was not normalised by the interviewees but accepted or tolerated if users adhered to certain conventions or social rules. In particular, school attendees were critical of the lifestyles and social activities of 'hard' drug and chaotic users. They thought that heroin was not easy to obtain and that its use was associated with being older and existing in 'a different social world'. There is support for this opinion from a survey of young people referred from the area to addiction services.

The young people had clear opinions about the drugs education they had received. They were especially sensitive to what they saw as adults' hypocrisy and were critical of 'scare story' approaches to education. In line with findings in the USA, they recommended that education should be more interactive and conducted away from school premises and by people with first- or second-hand experience.

Another recent qualitative survey shows the opinions of young people aboout the child and adolescent mental health services they had received. These opinions contribute to an agenda for workforce development and service design (Buston, 2002).

A strategic framework

Together We Stand (Williams & Richardson, 1995) proposed a four-tier strategic framework that is now well-established as the basis for developing child and adolescent mental health services. *The Substance of Young Needs* (Williams *et al*, 1996) developed a similar functional tiered strategic framework to capture: the wide spectrum of services required by young people who use or misuse substances; the content and levels of training required by staff; and the capabilities and variations in dedicated specialisation required to deliver a sufficiently comprehensive array of services. The tiers are:

Tier 1   universal, primary-level services;
Tier 2   youth-oriented services;
Tier 3   services provided by teams that specialise in treating young people who misuse substances;
Tier 4   very specialised services for young people who misuse substances.

The tiered concept is a flexible and dynamic strategic approach that provides a framework within which to conceptualise the functions of comprehensive services and relationships between their commissioners and providers. It emphasises activities rather than the disciplines of professionals and promotes integration between sectors, agencies and disciplines. The intention is to enable stakeholders to formulate integrated and comprehensive care plans for each young person and family, and avoid fitting children to what is available.

This framework allows commissioners in all sectors to negotiate and share: clear plans for comprehensive services; the gaps in current provision; plans for investment; better understanding of inter-organisational relationships; and coordination of the work of relevant agencies. It allows service providers:

* to generate common goals and networks;
* to collaborate to avoid fragmentation and maximise delivery of seamless, multi-component responses to people who have complex needs;
* to support each other to facilitate skill transfer, planned professional development, and training;
* to match young people's needs to the most appropriate interventions; and
* to agree the role and target populations for prevention and intervention.

A service model

This section brings together the influences summarised earlier in this chapter to develop a model for services for young people who use or misuse substances. We use the four-tier framework to bring the model together.

Tier 1

Description

Tier 1 is the front-line service to which all children and families have direct access. It consists of primary-level services provided by the health, education, social and voluntary sector services.

Staff

The professionals include teachers, staff of voluntary sector agencies, primary health care and school health services, and the police.

Activities

Already some practitioners are concerned with improving and maintaining health, while others are engaged in work that bears upon the risk factors and consequences of substance use and misuse. While some practitioners should be involved in delivering universal education programmes, others should be trained to deliver selective education targeted on those more at risk.

All the staff (see above) are well placed to recognise vulnerability and substance misuse and to provide simple assessments and interventions for young people and families, provided they receive the required training and support to do so from Tiers 2 and 3.

Examples

- Nurses in primary health care who provide well-adolescent clinics for those over 16 years old that improve recognition of vulnerability and provide advice on substances and health, including sexual health.
- School nurses who provide advice and information for parents and children who smoke tobacco.

Tier 2

Description

Tier 2 describes the first line of more specialised services, in which it is critical to identify vulnerable young people and provide early intervention programmes. Despite developments since 1996, very much more remains much to be done, as few areas yet have comprehensive Tier 2 services that are adequate to meet assessed need or the potential demand.

Staff

These services are offered by practitioners with some experience of and training for working with people who use or misuse substances, and some knowledge and skills related to working with young people. The range of practitioners is wide and should include the staff of the following: specialist child and adolescent mental health services; specialised voluntary sector youth services; paediatric and child health services; and youth offending teams. Additionally, certain primary health care practitioners, teachers and staff of the education support services who have a more specialised remit and training may have sufficient skills to discharge some functions of this tier.

Activities

This tier should be concerned with:

- reducing risk and vulnerability;
- reintegrating young people into mainstream services as well as maintaining them in generic services (e.g. school);
- providing targeted and indicated programmes;
- providing training, support and consultation to practitioners who deliver Tier 1 functions or activities.

Often, by virtue of being more vulnerable, the young people concerned require several interventions provided by different agencies. It is important that these interventions are provided according to the severity and range of an individual's problems and that responses to that individual's education, health and social problems are integrated within purposeful care plans. This requires:

- active integration of service responses;
- outreach services to engage young people who are excluded or who exclude themselves (e.g. homeless people and truants);
- services for young people and families in crisis;
- school liaison services;
- attention to the mental health needs of young people and their families; and
- services that can provide individual counselling as well as practical support.

Examples

Services in some areas have developed posts for young people's workers to work within existing addiction services for adults or, in others, within primary health care or community mental health teams. In other instances, workers with a specialist role and training are located in separate organisations (e.g. drugs workers attached to youth offending teams).

Other places have developed 'one-stop shops' to offer a broad approach that fosters development of a wide range of appropriate interventions and styles; together, the staff have a range of specialised skills. An example is of a service that employs Bangladeshi staff to act as mentors with a view to improving the accessibility and cultural diversity of substance misuse services.

Tier 3

Description

Some young people require rather more specialised interventions provided by services that have a core role in responding to young people who misuse substances and that are staffed by professionals with special training. Some of the young misusers requiring Tier 3 levels of care will have serious developmental, health, educational and social problems, and others may have substance misuse disorders that require specialist addiction services.

Current evidence provides powerful reasons why specialist services for young people who misuse substances should have close working relationships with mental health teams. The two services should come together to develop joint programmes and to ensure the competence and training of staff in matters relating to both substance misuse and young people's mental health.

Staff

Tier 3 is provided by multi-disciplinary teams of staff who are specifically trained and skilled for work with young people who misuse substances or who have substance misuse syndromes. Work at this level requires collaboration between child and adolescent mental health, addiction, education, paediatric, social and voluntary sector services and there are many organisational possibilities. One method is to create new teams; another approach is to draw on a variety of agencies to gather the appropriate skills around particular young people and the problems they present on a needs-led, case-managed basis; and a third way is to create clinical networks or 'virtual teams'. Together, the teams should be able to assess and manage the complex needs of young people who have more serious disorders.

Activities

The young people who are likely to require assessment and intervention at Tier 3 are also likely to have experienced multiple risk factors, social exclusion and comorbidity. The essential requirement is for collaboration between practitioners to produce a high degree of aggregate competence that results in systems that are capable of responding to multiple problems of high complexity.

Examples

In recent years, there have been some developments of teams at this level of capability in the UK. Examples include services (which ordinarily provide Tier 2 functions) in which the core team is augmented by contracted time (for the provision of Tier 3 services) provided by: an addiction psychiatrist; a child and adolescent psychiatrist; a psychologist; nurses with child mental health and addiction skills; and a teacher.

Tier 4

Description

The functions designated as being in Tier 4 are those very specialised ones that are not required in each area, but to which reliable access is needed for a very few patients. Tier 4 functions include those provided by in-patient and residential units, intensive day centres, specialised crisis placements, specialised housing or fostering, and formal multi-systemic therapies that may at times have a residential focus. The essence is of multi-component packages of care for young people with very complex needs for particular periods rather than necessarily particular settings (Gilvarry *et al*, 2001). There are major gaps in service provision for the relatively small numbers of young people who require services that offer this intensity or specialisation of provision. Particularly, there has been little development of purpose-specific residential units for young people who, for example, require detoxification.

Staff

The staff required are of similarly diverse backgrounds and require similarly specialised training and environments as those who work in Tier 3. If the latter is a residential unit, experience of work in such a setting is core, as is, for some, management of young people with dependence and severe substance use disorders.

Activities

In-patient and residential settings may be more appropriate for: young people who have more serious substance use disorders together with significant comorbid problems; those at risk of significant withdrawal syndromes; and young people who have failed to respond to community-based interventions. These residential and day units should provide intensive and structured multi-component programmes for young people with serious or multiple problems.

Some interventions (e.g. multi-systemic therapies) are resource and contact intensive and, therefore, expensive. However, they are beginning to show positive results when used with very troubled adolescents who have multiple needs (e.g. young offenders with substance misuse) (Henggeler *et al*, 1998).

Examples

The number of in-patient or other residential facilities dedicated to young people is tiny. In a number of places, solutions have been sought by bringing expertise from specialist child and adolescent mental health services and specialist addiction services (Tier 3 activities) together with existing in-patient facilities to deliver focused work of high intensity for short periods with particular people. Other facilities that could be considered for use in this way include day units, forensic mental health in-patient units, specialised crisis placements, specialised housing and certain foster placements.

Lessons from experience

Whenever possible, any interventions should be delivered and managed by Tiers 1 and 2, as this allows a broader approach, greater continuity and less stigmatisation, and 'normalises' the situation for young people and their families. Involving young people in designing and delivering the services promotes their credibility.

Presently, very many more young people are in need than can be referred to Tier 2. Rather than their needs, it is likely that the burden experienced by families and staff delivering Tier 1 is the main feature that distinguishes those young people who are referred to more specialised services from those who are not. Resolution of this problem requires: substantial development of Tier 2, 3 and 4 functions; improved support and training for Tier 1; and a greater range of services in Tier 2, to include a great many more centres to which young people may refer themselves.

The risk of employing single staff within teams that have other functions is that they can become isolated and suffer skill dilution or loss of focus on their primary tasks. Small numbers of practitioners attached to services for adults may not be able to sustain a child-centred focus or multi-disciplinary and multi-agency work. So it is important that, where staff are out-posted as single practitioners, they are also part of a network of staff with similar training and tasks, and are enabled to link with colleagues who provide Tier 3 services. This aids the flow of referrals, improves working practices and allows staff to benefit from clinical supervision. Networks of out-posted practitioners can create a critical mass of expertise and competence that is capable of offering support to other generic workers in child care and child health systems.

Decisions about the best setting in which to offer intervention turn on a number of factors, including: the severity of the substance problems and any associated psychiatric and physical problems; the ability of each young person to care for himself or herself; the nature and intensity of the treatments required; responses to past treatments; the settings available; and the preferences of each family and child.

Planning, implementation and organisational development

A number of other matters require attention when designing and implementing services. Organisational and staff development plans created by local agencies are vital parts of the comprehensive model. National programmes are also required.

Workforce issues

Much more could be done to help young people who are at risk of progressing to substance misuse or who already have problems that stem from it, if there were more and better-trained people in UK services. Although there is much more to be learned from research and, realistically, limitations to what can be done to resolve many situations, the most significant problems now do not lie in knowledge or potential professional capability but rather in service capacity.

This book points to the huge agenda for generating and training the staff required. Also, there is abundant evidence from this book that the world in which we ask staff to function is characterised by complexity and uncertainty, and that some decisions that practitioners are required to make pose significant professional and personal challenges. Staff require effective systems of education, mentoring and reflective supervision if they are to cope well, learn from their experiences and assist their patients maximally (Williams, 2002). Therefore, none of the agencies can afford to assume that creating a plan to develop services and finding money to finance it are sufficient. The general risks of employers not taking seriously the workforce issues could well be related to a flurry of literature concerning the poor morale of professionals (see Edwards *et al*, 2002 for an entry point). No plan can be considered to be adequate without a workforce development strategy that deals forthrightly and realistically with recruitment and retention of staff and their training and supervision.

Service culture

Similarly, there are a number of organisational matters that must be resolved to facilitate the execution of desirable care plans. In the main, these matters relate to the culture of the organisations that deliver services.

Valuing young people, child protection and information sharing

Primacy must be given to recognising that these services are for minors. The Carlile review (National Assembly for Wales, 2002) has shown the importance of creating an organisational culture that values and protects young people and allows proper exchange of information on a verified need-to-know basis. Advocacy services should be integral to substance misuse services.

We recognise that some agencies will find moving from a culture with high boundaries around confidentiality to the kind of culture we describe here is a challenge and the work required to support and maintain it should not be underestimated.

Families as well as individuals

Similarly, awareness of the needs of families as well as individuals is key. While we believe that a focus on young people must not be lost, and their needs have primacy when all else fails, our services must also be able to support families, as failure to resolve crucial problems for adults may limit achievements with their children. This calls for improved collaboration between services for adults and those for children.

Collaboration

Good inter-agency collaboration is essential to ensuring continuity and coordination of care. A case management system can ensure that care is prompt and continuous, appropriate and delivered in settings that are accessible and appropriate for children, adolescents and their families. The key is not only continuity of care within a particular agency but also coordination of care and interventions across the agencies involved.

Experience suggests that collaboration across departmental and agency boundaries may falter all too easily. Over a number of years, work conducted by the Dartington Social Research Unit has shown that these recurrent problems stem from differences in agencies and the professions relating to: theoretical approaches to the work; organisational structure and function; definitions of the client group; and perceptions of need, risk and the purposes of the services. A review of the literature by Bullock & Little (1999) provides an entry point to some of Dartington's research (also see Little & Bullock, 2004). The qualitative work that is taking place in Wales confirms the importance of these issues to delivering effective care for young people who misuse substances.

Projects undertaken to find solutions show that there can be no replacement for hard work and that the challenges to inter-agency working must be resolved before lasting progress can be made. The solutions require longer-term stability of organisational structures and relationships between key players. Better integration between the tiers and collaboration between different agencies working within the same tier can be promoted by: effective care planning; joint training; and developing a shared language that crosses professional and agency boundaries. The Welsh Institute for Health and Social Care has analysed the problems and developed a three-component approach to improving collaboration within services and across agency boundaries (Williams & Salmon, 2002)

The challenge for the future

In this chapter, we have sought to bring together the contents of the book to think about how services for young people who use and misuse substances might be designed. We have presented a comprehensive approach that is consistent with policy, developed through strategy and informed by evidence from research, young people, experience and professional practice.

Our key conclusion is that services must deal with people and the full range of their problems – not just their symptoms or syndromes. The corollary is the importance of improving collaboration between all the care sectors. This integrated approach is reflected in the strategic intent (aims and objectives) and the principles. Our evidence-based approach to design is held together with the other features of our model by a four-tier strategic framework.

It is clear that the field has moved rapidly in the past decade in the UK, yet there remains a huge amount to do before we have comprehensive services. EBSD takes history into account by recognising that designs are not written on a clean sheet. There are important background challenges to solve including: previous absence of strategy; current services being unrelated to need; achieving the financial long-termism that is required to sustain and develop services; and recruiting, retaining, properly training and valuing a substantially increased staff. EBSD brings these vital matters into conjunction with evidence from people, science and the humanities. Strategic and operational leadership is required to ensure that we are able to use what we know and our skills to improve services for young people.

References

Aarons, G. A., Brown, S. A., Hough, R. L., *et al* (2001) Prevalence of adolescent substance use disorders across five sectors of care. *Journal of the American Academy of Child and Adolescent Psychiatry*, **40**, 419–426.

American Academy of Pediatrics Commission on Substance Misuse (2001) Alcohol use and abuse: a pediatric concern. *Pediatrics*, **108**, 185–189.

Barton, A. & Quinn, C. (2001) The supremacy of joined-up workings: a Pandora's box for organisational identity. *Public Policy and Administration*, **16**, 49–62.

Barton, H., Davey, I., Street, E., *et al* (2002) Lot 3. Mental health in childhood, children and young people who have mental health problems and mental disorders and mental health services for young people. Internet: Papers of the Health and Social Services Committee of the National Assembly for Wales for 25 April 2002, at http://www.wales.gov.uk

Becker, H. S. (1991) *Outsiders: Studies in the Sociology of Deviance*. New York: Free Press.

Belcher, H. & Schinitzly, H. (1998) Substance abuse in children: prediction, protection and prevention. *Archives of Paediatric and Adolescent Medicine*, **152**, 952–960.

Bonomo, Y., Coffey, C., Wolfe, R., *et al* (2001) Adverse outcomes of alcohol use in adolescents. *Addiction*, **96**, 1485–1496.

Brown, S. A., Amico, A. J. D., McCarthy, D. M., *et al* (2001) Four-year outcomes from adolescent alcohol and drug treatment. *Journal of Studies on Alcohol*, **62**, 381–388.

Bullock, R. & Little, M. (1999) The interface between social and health services for children and adolescent persons. *Current Opinion in Psychiatry*, **12**, 421–424.

Bushell, H. D., Crome, I. & Williams, R. J. W. (2002) How can risk be related to interventions for young people who misuse substances? *Current Opinion in Psychiatry*, **15**, 355–360.

Buston, K. (2002) Adolescents with mental health problems: what do they say about health services? *Journal of Adolescence*, **25**, 231–242.

Byrne, P., Jones, S. & Adamson, D. (2002). Personal communication of unpublished research data. Pontypridd: University of Glamorgan.

Central Drugs Coordination Unit (1999) *To Build a Better Britain: The Government's Ten Year Strategy for Tackling Drug Misuse*. London: Cabinet Office.

Dale-Perera, A., Hamilton, C., Evans, K., *et al* (1999) *Young People and Drugs: Policy Guidance for Drug Interventions*. London: Standing Conference on Drug Abuse, Children's Legal Centre.

Department of Health, Department for Education and Employment & Home Office (2000) *Framework for the Assessment of Children in Need and their Families*. London: The Stationery Office.

Edwards, E., Kornacki, M. J. & Silversin, J. (2002) Unhappy doctors: what are the causes and what can be done? *British Medical Journal*, **324**, 835–838.

Eggert, L. L., Thompson, E. A., Herting, J. R., *et al* (1994) Preventing adolescent drug abuse and high school drop-out through an intensive school based social network development programme. *American Journal of Health Promotion*, **8**, 202–215.

Farrell, M. & Strang, J. (1998) Editorial. Britain's new strategy for tackling drugs misuse shows a welcome emphasis on evidence. *British Medical Journal*, **316**, 1399–1400.

Ferdinand, R. F., Blum, M. & Verhulst, F. C. (2001) Psychopathology in adolescence predicts substance use in young adulthood. *Addiction*, **96**, 861–870.

Fulford, K. W. M. & Williams, R. (2003) Values-based child and adolescent mental health services? *Current Opinion in Psychiatry*, **16**, 369–376.

Giancola, P. R. & Parker, A. M. (2001) A six year prospective study of pathways toward drug use in adolescent boys with and without a family history of a substance use disorder. *Journal of Studies on Alcohol*, **62**, 166–178.

Gilvarry, E., Christian, J., Crome, I., *et al* (2001) *The Substance of Young Needs: Review 2001*. London: Health Advisory Service.

Goldberg, D. (2002) From a lecture given by Professor Sir David Goldberg in Cardiff in March 2002.

Goulden, C. & Sondhi, A. (2001) *At the Margins: Drug Use by Vulnerable Young People in the 1998/99 Youth Lifestyles Survey*. Home Office Research Study 228. London: Home Office Research, Development and Statistics Directorate.

Grella, C. E., Hser, Y-I., Joshi, V., *et al* (2001) Drug treatment outcomes for adolescents with comorbid mental and substance use disorders. *Journal of Nervous and Mental Disease*, **189**, 384–392.

Henggeler, S., Schoenwald, S., Borduin, C., *et al* (1998) *Multisystemic Treatment of Antisocial Behaviour in Children and Adolescents*. New York: Guilford Press.

Juang, L. P. & Silbereisen, R. K. (2002) The relationship between adolescent academic capability beliefs, parenting and school grades. *Journal of Adolescence*, **25**, 3–18.

Kumpfer, K. L., Molgaard, V. & Spoth, R. (1996) The 'Strenghtening Families Program' for the prevention of delinquency and drug use. In *Preventing Childhood Disorders, Substance Abuse and Delinquency* (eds R. Peters & R. McMahon), pp. 242–267. Thousand Oaks, CA: Sage.

Kuperman, S., Schlosser, S. S., Kramer, J. R., *et al* (2001) Risk domains associated with an adolescent alcohol dependence diagnosis. *Addiction*, **96**, 629–636.

Little, M. & Bullock, R. (2004) Administrative frameworks and services for very difficult adolescents in England. In *Forensic Adolescent Psychiatry* (eds S. Bailey & M. Dolan). London: Arnold, in press.

Miller, P. & Plant, M. (1996) Drinking, smoking and illicit drug use among 15 and 16 year olds in the United Kingdom. *British Medical Journal*, **313**, 394–397.

Mullen, L. & Barry, J. (2001) An analysis of 15–19 year-old first attenders at the Dublin Needle Exchange, 1990–97. *Addiction*, **96**, 251–258.

National Assembly for Wales (2000a) *Children and Young People: A Framework for Partnership*. Cardiff: National Assembly for Wales.

—— (2000b) *Tackling Substance Misuse in Wales: A Partnership Approach*. Cardiff: National Assembly for Wales.

—— (2001) *Everybody's Business – Child and Adolescent Mental Health Services Strategy Document*. Cardiff: National Assembly for Wales.

—— (2002) *Too Serious a Thing – the Carlile Review*. Cardiff: National Assembly for Wales.

—— & Home Office (2001) *Framework for the Assessment of Children in Need and Their Families*. London: The Stationery Office

Pedersen, W., Mastekaasa, A. & Wichtrom, L. (2001) Conduct problems and early cannabis initiation: a longitudinal study of gender differences. *Addiction*, **96**, 415–431.

Rivers, S. M., Greenbaum, R. L. & Goldberg, E. (2001) Hospital-based adolescent substance abuse treatment: comorbidity, outcomes and gender. *Journal of Nervous and Mental Disease*, **189**, 229–237.

Social Exclusion Unit (2001) *Preventing Social Exclusion*. Report by the Social Exclusion Unit. At http://www.cabinet-office.gov.uk/seu/index.htm.

Spoth, R. L., Redmond, C. & Shin, C. (2001) Randomized trial of brief family interventions for general populations: adolescent substance use outcomes 4 years following baseline. *Journal of Consulting and Clinical Psychology*, **69**, 627–642.

Sussman, S. (1996) Development of a school based drug abuse prevention curriculum for high risk youths. *Journal of Psychoactive Drugs*, **28**, 169–182.

Sutherland, I. & Shepherd, J. P. (2002) Adolescents' beliefs about future substance use: a comparison of current users and non-users of cigarettes, alcohol and illicit drugs. *Journal of Adolescence*, **25**, 169–181

Tudor Hart, J. (1971) The inverse care law. *Lancet, i,* 405–412.

Warner, M. & Furnish, S. (2002) Towards coherent policy and practice in Alzheimer's disease across the EU. In *Alzheimer's Disease – Policy and Practice Across Europe* (eds M. Warner, S. Furnish, M. Longley, *et al*). Abingdon: Radcliffe Medical Press.

Weinberg, N., Rahdert, E., Colliver, J. *et al* (1998) Adolescent substance abuse: a review of the past 10 years. *Journal of the American Academy of Child and Adolescent Psychiatry,* **37,** 252–261.

Williams, R. (2002) Complexity, uncertainty and decision-making in an evidence-based world. *Current Opinion in Psychiatry,* **15,** 343–347.

—— & Richardson, G. (eds) (1995) *Together We Stand – The Commissioning, Role and Management of Child and Adolescent Mental Health Services.* London: HMSO, Health Advisory Service.

—— & Salmon, G. (2002) Collaboration in commissioning and delivering child and adolescent mental health services. *Current Opinion in Psychiatry,* **15,** 349–353.

——, Christian, J., Gay, M., *et al* (eds) (1996) *The Substance of Young Needs: Commissioning and Providing Services for Children and Young People Who Use and Misuse Substances.* London: HMSO, Health Advisory Service.

Winters, K. C. (1999) *Treatment of Adolescents with Substance Use Disorders: Treatment Improvement Protocol (TIP) Series 32.* US Department of Health and Human Services publication no. (SMA) 99–3283. Rockville, MD: US Department of Health and Human Services.

Zeitlin, H. (1999) Psychiatric comorbidity with substance misuse in children and teenagers. *Drug and Alcohol Dependence,* **55,** 225–234.

Index

Compiled by Linda English